Neck Complaints

THE MOST COMMON COMPLAINTS SERIES

Headache
Egilius L. H. Spierings

Confusion
Karl E. Misulis and Terri Edwards-Lee

Neck Complaints
Michael Ronthal

Neck
Complaints

Michael Ronthal, MbBCh, FRCP

*Associate Professor of Neurology, Harvard Medical School,
Boston; Deputy Chief of Neurology, Beth Israel Deaconess
Medical Center, Boston*

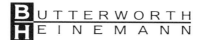

Boston   Oxford   Auckland   Johannesburg   Melbourne   New Delhi

Library of Congress Cataloging-in-Publication Data
Ronthal, Michael, 1938-
    Neck Complaints / Michael Ronthal.
        p.   cm. -- (The most common complaints)
    Includes bibliographical references and index.
    ISBN 0-7506-7156-4 ✔
    1. Neck pain. 2. Neck--Care and hygiene. I. Title. II. Series.
    [DNLM: 1. Neck Pain. 2. Neck Injuries. 3. Spinal Osteophytosis.
WE 708 R774n 2000]
RD763.R66 2000
617.5'3--dc21
DNLM/DLC
for Library of Congress   99-37382
                                                                          CIP

British Library Cataloguing-in-Publication Data
A catalogue record for this book is available from the British Library.

The publisher offers special discounts on bulk orders of this book.

For information, please contact:
Manager of Special Sales   For information on all
Butterworth–Heinemann   Butterworth–Heinemann
225 Wildwood Avenue   publications available, contact
Woburn, MA 01801-2041   our World Wide Web home
Tel: 781-904-2500   page at: http://www.bh.com
Fax: 781-904-2620

10 9 8 7 6 5 4 3 2 1

Printed in the United States of America

*For my wife, Berenice, who over the years
has patiently waited for me to put down the pen,
now a word processor! My true friend.*

Contents

Preface

Complaints related to the cervical spine are among the most common presenting symptoms seen by clinical neurologists. Patients with symptoms relating to the neck also constitute a significant fraction of primary care practice, and, unless handled with dexterity, continue to return with ongoing symptoms, causing both patient and physician frustration. It is for this reason that this volume is included in *The Most Common Complaints* repertoire.

Diagnoses range from simple muscle contraction headache in anxious and tense individuals to cervical spondylosis with significant cervical stenosis and cord compression requiring decompressive surgery. The trick is to make an accurate diagnosis and to know when to investigate further by way of imaging and when to pursue a conservative, supportive role that also contains symptoms. Patients are frequently convinced that they have a brain tumor, and the treating physician is often infected with the same anxiety, leading to costly and unnecessary tests. Especially in our current cost-conscious climate, a return to the "clinical method," which embraces an accurate physical examination and a measured approach to management, is the order of the day. "Shotgun" and ill-considered investigation is not cost-effective and often fails to make the diagnosis. A "rule-out" approach is neither frugal nor effective. If the lessons of this book result in the clinical method practice approach, the effort expended in writing it will be adequately rewarded.

This preface would not be complete without a few words in remembrance of my mentor, Norman Geschwind. As a young attending physician, I presented case after case—all with unusual physical signs and symptoms suggesting weird and wonderful esoteric diagnoses. Norman would listen carefully to my argument, shake his head, wave his hand, and answer, "spondylosis." Of course he was always right—a good lesson, and well learned.

The Introduction reviews James Parkinson's 1817 essay on the "shaking palsy"—which, at first glance, one would think has nothing to do with cervical spondylosis—all the way to current practice.

Truth to tell, our knowledge of the pathophysiology of the clinical syndromes described is incomplete, and the "best" treatments have never been tested in prospective controlled trials. No controlled trials of treatment of cervical spondylosis or whiplash injury of the neck, either conservatively or by way of surgery, exist. Although the diagnostic signs and symptoms described herein are based on a solid clinical foundation and will stand the test of time, the treatments suggested are simply a personal "best and current practice."

I have been treating neck problems for more than 35 years and offer the benefit of my experience rather than a tested scientific approach. Drug treatment has evolved over the years—practitioners initially used amylobarbitone, then graduated to Librium, then Valium combined with tricyclics, and, more recently, selective serotonin uptake inhibitors—all based on patient response. To be sure, sometimes we are simply treating a somatic equivalent of depression, but most patients have organic problems, and if nothing else, we should be in the business of relieving pain. Large clinical practices are built by word of mouth of satisfied customers, not by the number of brain tumors diagnosed!

This approach has worked for me and I hope it will work for the reader in his or her practice.

M. R.

Historical Introduction

Evolution of modern concepts of the pathophysiology of spinal cord injury can be traced back as far as ancient Egypt and the Edwin Smith papyrus. In 1862, Smith purchased from Mustapha Aga, an Egyptian merchant living in Thebes, a 21½-column papyrus, which was subsequently given to the New York Historical Society and ultimately translated by Breasted in 1930. A case of cervical cord injury is described as follows: "One having a dislocation in a vertebra of his neck while he is unconscious of his two legs and his arms and his urine dribbles—an ailment not to be treated."

James Parkinson, in his essay on the shaking palsy (1817), gave excellent descriptions of patients with cervical radiculopathy. He believed that the symptoms of parkinsonism were due to "a diseased state of the medulla spinalis in that part which is contained in the canal, formed by the superior cervical vertebrae, and extending, as the disease proceeds, to the medulla oblongata." He observed that "the greater degree of mobility in that portion of the spine which is formed by the superior cervical vertebrae, must render it, and the contained parts, liable to injury from sudden distortions." He described patient A. B., who was "subject to rheumatic affection of the deltoid muscle, had felt the usual inconveniences from it for two or three days; but at night found the pain had extended down the arm, along the inside of the forearm, and on the sides of the fingers, in which a continuous tingling was felt. The pain, without being extremely intense, was such as effectually to prevent sleep: and seemed to follow the course of the brachial nerve." The patient's symptoms were relieved in 4 or 5 days by the following treatment: "Blood was taken from the back part of the neck by cupping; hot fomentations were applied for about the space of an hour, when the upper part of the back of the neck was covered with a blister, perspiration was freely induced by two or three small doses of antimonials, and the following morning the bowels were evacuated by an appropriate dose of calomel." The patient improved because of, or in spite of, the treatment—an allegation that might be aimed at many modern-day treatments and nostrums!

John Kearsley Mitchell (S. Weir Mitchell's father) wrote about nervous system consequences of noncarious spondylitis or spondylosis (1831), but his index case is not convincing—he described a woman who had had pains in the neck, which subsided as she developed severe wrist pain associated with redness, tumefaction, and heat.

C. A. Key (1838), in *Guy's Hospital Reports*, accurately described a spondylotic bar at autopsy: "the obstruction was shown to be occasioned by a projection of the intervertebral substance, or rather the posterior ligament of the spine, which was thickened and presented a firm ridge, which had lessened the diameter of the canal by nearly a third."

Romberg, in his 1840 text, *A Manual of the Nervous Diseases of Man*, described cervical neuralgia. He commented, "These varieties of neuralgia are very enduring; they continue for years; and the effect of remedies is very doubtful. Remissions may take place under the most opposite treatment." He suggested "steel"—that is, iron—as a treatment, and recommended warm baths and douches at Wiesbaden and Aix-la-Chapelle but denounced cold, wet sheets.

Vladimir von Bechterew in 1893 described patients with cord or root dysfunction, or both, which he thought was due to a single entity characterized more or less by immobility of the spinal column or a part of it, without any particular pain being produced by percussion of the spinal column or bending. He entitled his paper *Rigidity and Curvature of the Vertebral Column as a Special Form of Disease*.

Victor Horsley, the "father of brain surgery," at least in Britain, performed the first successful surgery for cervical spondylosis in 1892. The patient, under the influence of alcohol, fell off his van, developed severe right brachialgia, and, 2 weeks later, his arms weakened. Over the next 2 months, he became paraparetic with loss of sphincter control. Horsley performed a laminectomy at C6 and found the cord to be compressed by a transverse ridge projecting backward from the body of the vertebra. The patient recovered completely within a year.

Sir William Gowers (1892), a contemporary of Horsley at Queen Square Hospital in London, described exostoses growing from the vertebral bodies into the spinal canal, which might compress cord or nerves, but thought they were extremely rare.

In 1911, Pearce Bailey and Luis Casamajor, with the help of improving roentgenography, discussed osteoarthritis of the spine and described five patients with cervical radiculopathy. They thought that the primary pathology was a thinning of the intervertebral disks, and that this led to changes in the bodies of the vertebrae, including bony overgrowth.

Elliot, in 1926, described how radicular symptoms might be caused by narrowing of the intervertebral foramina. In 1928, Stookey described cord and root compression by "ventral extra dural chondromas," and 1 year later, Schmorl described the anatomy and pathology of the intervertebral disk protrusion. The concept of chondroma, however, was strengthened by the work of Elsberg, who recorded in a paper on extradural tumors that 7 of 46 such tumors were chondromas. In 1932, Peet and Echols reported that the chondroma of previous authors was really a protrusion of the intervertebral disk. Microscopically, they saw a normal nucleus pulposus.

At the New England Surgical Society meeting in Boston in September of 1933, Mixter and Barr reported on their experience using surgery for the treatment of disk disease. Myelography demonstrated cervical blocks in four patients, laminectomy was done in three, all of whom were "much improved." The paper was published in *The New England Journal of Medicine* in 1934 but is best remembered for its description of the lumbar disk disease.

Numerous other contributions followed, only some of which are highlighted. In 1948, Bull correlated the radiology of osteophytes at the neurocentral joints of Luschka invading the intervertebral foramen with radicular symptoms but pointed out that the absence of osteophytes did not exclude pressure on the nerve due to periarticular soft tissue swelling, invisible on plain x-rays. Brain, in the same year, drew a distinction between acute, often traumatic, disk protrusion causing neurologic signs and symptoms, and chronic compression associated with osteophyte growth.

In 1951, Frykholm distinguished nuclear herniation from annular protrusion. The former is originally soft but may be transformed into a cartilaginous mass, which may calcify. The latter is fibrocartilaginous but gradually calcifies. He also suggested that root sleeve fibrosis might cause root compression. In 1953, Taylor pointed out that the cord could also be compressed by hypertrophy or buckling of the ligamentum flavum.

Pallis, Jones, and Spillane (1954) stressed spondylosis is common. They found that 50% of people older than 50 years, and 75% of people older than 65 years, had typical radiologic changes of cervical spondylosis. Forty percent of people older than 50 years have some limitation of neck movement, and 60% have some neurologic abnormality if examined carefully.

FURTHER READING

Bailey P, Casamajor L. Osteo-arthritis of the spine as a cause of compression of the spinal cord and its roots: with reports of five cases. J Nerv Ment Dis 1911;38:588.

Bull JWD. Discussion on rupture of the intervertebral disc in the cervical region. Proc R Soc Med 1948;41:513.

Frykholm R. Cervical nerve root compression resulting from disc degeneration and root sleeve fibrosis. A clinical investigation. Acta Chir Scand 1951;Suppl 160.

Gowers WR. Disease of the Nervous System (2nd ed), Vol.1. London: Churchill 1892;260.

Mixter WJ, Barr JS. Rupture of the intervertebral disk with involvement of the spinal canal. N Engl J Med 1934;211:210.

Pallis CA, Jones AM, Spillane JD. Cervical spondylosis. Brain 1954;77:274.

Parkinson J (1817). An Essay on the Shaking Palsy. London: Sherwood, Neely and Jones, 1817.

Neck Pain and Headache

A 57-year-old man complained of intermittent headache for 3 weeks. The pain was described as a
constant, aching bifrontal pain that was worse in the
morning on arising, settled as the morning wore on,
and became worse again in the evening. No specific
aggravating or relieving features were present.
Although he felt slightly off balance at times, no true
vertigo was present. He had experienced some
tightness and stiffness in his neck and tingling in his
right arm. He denied weakness and had no long-
tract symptoms. On examination, neck rotation to
the right and left was limited by approximately 20
degrees. A good deal of posterior cervical muscle
spasm and tenderness was present. No weakness
or sensory loss was present in the upper limbs, but

the biceps reflexes were absent, and the triceps reflexes were brisk. No long-tract signs were present in the lower limbs.

DISCUSSION

Pain associated with cervical spondylosis is referred from pain-sensitive structures in the neck. These structures include the muscles surrounding the vertebral column, sensory nerves and roots, bone, dura, and disks. Pathology at any of these sites can be the origin of local neck pain or referred pain. A painful, stiff neck or referred muscle contraction headache is the most common symptom of early cervical spondylosis.

Neck muscle spasm in cervical spondylosis can be regarded as a splinting mechanism to prevent movement of the neck. The spasm is a reflex muscle contraction triggered by irritation of pain-sensitive structures. In young patients without cervical spondylosis, the spasm is usually generated by emotional stress or tension. Muscles in continuous spasm produce lactic acid via anaerobic metabolism, which in turn stimulates pain receptors. Pain is transmitted to the central nervous system via sensory cervical nerve roots and the ascending central pathways, which converge with the pathways from the trigeminal nerve so that the pain can be referred anteriorly to trigeminal territory or to the back of the neck and back of the head in C2 distribution. Pain can also be referred to the ears via C3 connections, and pain just below and behind the ear lobe is a classical symptom of C1-C2 subluxation in rheumatoid arthritis.

SYMPTOMS

The pain or headache is often described as a tightness around the head, a squeezing or bursting sensation, or sometimes a feeling of pressure on the top of the head. The patient may or may not be aware of tightness and stiffness in the neck. The cause of pain is often thought to be an intracranial process, resulting in an unnecessary imaging study of the brain as the first diagnostic procedure.

The stiff neck and headache syndrome is often worse in the morning on arising. The reason may be that muscles become lax and the neck is unprotected during sleep, and pain-sensitive structures are irritated during tossing and turning or when the neck is stretched in awkward positions, resulting in more spasm and pain. Providing better neck support during sleep with hard pillows or a cervical collar frequently relieves the symptoms.

PHYSICAL SIGNS

The cardinal sign of cervical spondylosis is restriction of normal neck movement. This sign is best tested for by passive or active neck rotation. Normally, the neck should rotate so that the chin is virtually over the point of the shoulder; any restriction of movement to this landmark denotes reduced range of motion and establishes the diagnosis. In cases of acute, severe neck pain from any cause, however, range of motion is restricted voluntarily to minimize pain, and true spondylosis may not be present at all.

In patients with headache, palpation of the posterior cervical muscles reveals tight, tender muscles in spasm. Gentle massage of the neck muscle may relieve the headache, albeit temporarily, but demonstration of this sign is reassuring for both the physician and patient.

The finding of root or long-tract signs supports the diagnosis of spondylosis but is not necessary to make it.

TREATMENT

No adequate controlled trials of treatment have been reported; what follows is the author's personal approach to treatment.

Physical measures such as local heat, firm pillows, and sleeping in a collar should be tried first. Continuous use of a collar for 1 or 2 weeks is sometimes necessary. Physical therapy is useful, provided that the therapist is gentle and uses only massage, local heat, and perhaps ultrasound. Neck exercises usually exacerbate the problem and have no long-term benefit.

Some authors have reported benefit from acupuncture.

Chiropractic manipulation is mentioned only to condemn it; manipulation of the neck is dangerous. Reported complications of chiropractic manipulation include posterior arterial circulation thrombosis and dissection, subluxation and even fractures of the vertebrae, and spinal epidural hematoma. The only published randomized controlled trial did not demonstrate that manipulation was significantly helpful.

If the above measures fail, treatment is escalated to drug therapy. Any over-the-counter analgesic should be used as a first step. Nonsteroidal anti-inflammatory agents are good analgesics but play no special role in treating the headache and muscle spasm of cervical spondylosis and may be contraindicated in patients with upper gastrointestinal pathology. A muscle relaxant drug is usually combined with an antidepressant for treatment of chronic pain. I prefer diazepam, 2 mg three times a day, with paroxetine, 20 mg daily. Occasionally, in the absence of a response to this treatment, an epidural steroid injection should be considered. It provides temporary relief of pain in approximately 65% of patients.

FURTHER READING

Assendelft WJ, Bouter LM, Knipschild PG, Bouter SM. Complications of spinal manipulation: a comprehensive review of the literature. J Fam Pract 1996;42:475.

Barghout JA, Koes BW, Bouter LM. The clinical course and prognostic factors of non-specific neck pain: a systematic review. Pain 1998;77:1.

David J, Modi S, Aluko AA, et al. Chronic neck pain: a comparison of acupuncture treatment and physiotherapy. Br J Rheumatol 1998;37:1118.

Lee KP, Carlini WG, McCormick GF, Albers GW. Neurologic complications following chiropractic manipulation: a survey of California neurologists. Neurology 1995;45:1213.

Powell FC, Hanigan WC, Olivero WC. A risk/benefit analysis of spinal manipulation therapy for the relief of lumbar or cervical pain. Neurosurgery 1993;33:73.

Swezey RC. Chronic neck pain. Rheum Dis Clin North Am 1996;22:411.

Neurologic Symptoms

ROOT SYMPTOMS

Because the cervical nerve roots contain both motor and sensory fibers, the symptoms of nerve root irritation may be considered in terms of those arising in both afferent and efferent pathways.

Sensory Symptoms

Classic nerve root pain is sharp and lancinating, radiating down one or both upper limbs. It may be triggered, modified, or aggravated by neck movement and may be acute or subacute. Referred pain from irritation of the fifth cervical root is felt over the deltoid; pain referred from the sixth nerve root radiates to the forearm and thumb. Occasionally, anterior chest pain due to irritation of the fourth cervical root is misdiagnosed as coronary pain. Usually, however, the pain is described as anything from a mild, diffuse ache to a severe, diffuse brachialgia with no specific radiation. The patient may complain of numbness or tingling of the fingers. These symptoms have their origin in the small, slowly conducting pain and temperature fibers.

Symptoms arising from the fast conducting sensory system are rarely seen in cervical spondylosis. The symptoms consist of deep, aching, boring pain, or a feeling of squeezing at the wrist, as if the patient were wearing a tight elastic band. At times, the patient complains that the skin of the fingers feels too tight. These symptoms are probably not root in origin but more likely are posterior column tract–related and usually correlate with very high pathology in the cervical spine, even as high as the cranio-vertebral junction area, an extremely unusual site for cervical spondylosis. The presence of these symptoms therefore prompts imaging to search for pathology other than simple spondylosis.

Brachialgia aggravated by movement of peripheral joints suggests a local or rheumatologic cause and is not neurologic in origin. The most common rheumatologic complications of cervical spondylosis are shoulder bursitis and tendonitis. Although both can cause brachialgia, the clue to the diagnosis is aggravation of the pain by movement at the shoulder: In tendonitis, a painful arc of abduction is often present, and in bursitis, the patient complains of pain on reaching backward. Shoulder pain may also be part of the myofascial syndrome when palpable tender nodules are found in the posterior shoulder muscles.

Motor Symptoms

Patients rarely complain of weakness in proximal muscles. More often, they present with hand weakness and complain of difficulty with hand manipulations ("Things fall out of my hand"). Occasionally, complaints relate to triceps or deltoid weakness; thus, patients who exercise regularly may complain of difficulty doing push-ups because of elbow extension weakness, or they may complain of difficulty combing the hair because of shoulder weakness.

Muscle fasciculation may prompt the complaint of "live flesh."

SPINAL CORD SYMPTOMS

The spinal cord may be regarded as a major two-way highway and therefore produces symptoms and signs related to multiple afferent and efferent systems, both at the site of dysfunction and caudally to that site.

Motor long-tract dysfunction may result in a *gait disorder*, which can be secondary to weakness, spasticity, or loss of proprioception. The complaint may be of difficulty climbing stairs because of hip flexor weakness. Toe extensor weakness may cause the toes to catch on the stair lips; the patient may also catch his or her toe tips on ground irregularities or thick rugs, resulting in tripping. Spasticity causes feet scuffing and toe catching, and loss of proprioception produces an unsteady ataxic gait that is worse in the dark, so that falls may occur at night.

Sensory symptoms produced by deficits in ascending pathways are unusual but are occasionally the presenting complaint. Symptoms arising from dysfunction in the posterior column system have been discussed under Sensory Symptoms, earlier in this chapter; they are usually felt in the lower limbs. In addition, posterior cord irritation may result in a Lhermitte symptom: Flexion of the neck results in an electric shock–like pain in the arms, down the back, and even in the legs. Spinothalamic symptoms include numbness, tingling, itching, and occasionally sharp, superficial pain. These sensory symptoms may be referred to any cervical dermatome (root dysfunction) or somatic area caudal to the site of pathology (tract dysfunction). A burning, aching pain may occur in the legs and bears a superficial resemblance to sciatica (*sciatique cordonale*). Central cord dysfunction in the neck secondary to cervical spondylosis may result in loss of pain and temperature sensation in the upper limbs so that the patient has difficulty in gauging the temperature of water in the bathtub with the hands and complains of clumsy hands, yet temperature sensation in the feet is preserved.

Because the spinal tract of the trigeminal nerve descends into the upper cervical cord, high cord dysfunction occasionally results in a numb face, known as the *cervico-facial syndrome*.

BLADDER SYMPTOMS

Chronic myelopathy produces upper motor neuron symptoms caudal to the site of the lesion. The upper motor neuron bladder is spastic, small, and contracted. A low-capacity bladder results in frequency of micturition, and detrusor irritability causes urgency and urgency incontinence. Spinal cord dysfunction can also result in bladder dyssynergia; the detrusor contracts on a closed sphincter, and the patient experiences the usual, often urgent, desire to urinate but cannot initiate micturition.

Loss of bladder sensation is virtually unknown in cervical spondylosis, and a large deafferented atonic bladder usually suggests cauda equina pathology.

FURTHER READING

Heller JG. The syndromes of degenerative cervical disease. Orthop Clin North Am 1992;23:381.

Wilkinson, M (ed). Cervical Spondylosis: Its Early Diagnosis and Treatment (2nd ed). Philadelphia: Saunders, 1971.

Signs

A 64-year-old man complained of pain and stiffness in his neck with radiation to both shoulders and down the outer aspect of the left upper limb to the thumb. Neck movement aggravated his pain and the hand felt weak; he could not be more specific. He had a fluctuating, dull, constant aching headache, which radiated from the occipito-cervical region to the bifrontal region. For the previous 3 weeks he experienced frequency and urgency of micturition, but no incontinence had been present. He had no other long-tract symptoms. Examination revealed restricted neck movement, palpable posterior cervical muscle spasm with tenderness, and spasm in trapezius bilaterally. Mild weakness of finger extension, wrist extension, and triceps was present. The

lower fibers of pectoralis major were slightly weak.
The tendon reflexes were increased in all four limbs.
The plantar responses were flexor. Slight spasticity of
the lower limbs was present but no weakness. No
sensory deficit was present in the lower limbs.
Examination of the patient's shoes demonstrated
wear at the tips of the soles.

DISCUSSION

This patient has cervical spondylosis causing
painful restricted neck movement, and the symptoms and signs suggest C6-C7 radiculopathy.
Weakness or flabbiness of the lower fibers of pectoralis major indicates lower motor neuron weakness, and because the nerve to pectoralis branches
out close to the nerve root, weakness of pectoralis
localizes the pathology to root level. The mild spasticity and bladder symptoms indicate myelopathy
and suggest early cord compression.

ROOT SIGNS

Evidence of radiculopathy is found in approximately 90% of patients with cervical spondylosis,
usually bilaterally, although one side frequently
predominates.

Each root can be taken to supply specific muscle groups on the efferent side and to convey sensation from specific skin areas on the afferent side. Each motor segment is called a *myotome*, and each sensory segment is called a *dermatome*. Overlap in innervation of segments occurs, and each root supplies multiple muscles. If the clinician were to operate on a strict anatomic basis, localization of deficits to any particular single cervical root would be difficult. For clinical purposes, it is necessary to simplify the anatomy and functionally restrict the muscles supplied by the root in any particular segmental myotome (Table 3-1). Sensory loss is variable as well but in general conforms to the dermatomal map (Fig. 3-1). Compression or irritation of a nerve root can result in any combination of sensory symptoms, weakness, sensory loss, or reflex change of variable degree.

The finding of root signs allows for segmental localization in the neuraxis.

Wasting

As always, physical diagnosis begins with inspection. Wasting of muscle groups gives a clue to the root involved. Deltoid wasting is common in C5 root lesions. The sign is loss of the normal convex contour of the muscle, which is replaced by a concave contour or scalloping. Wasting of the small hand

Table 3-1. Main segmental innervation of the muscles of the upper limb

Segmental level	Muscle	Action
C5	Deltoid	Shoulder abduction
	Biceps/brachialis	Elbow flexion
C6	Extensor carpi radialis	Radial wrist extension
C6-C7	Triceps	Elbow extension
C7	Extensor digitorum	Finger extension
C8	Flexor digitorum	Finger flexion
T1	Interossei	Finger abduction/adduction
	Abductor digiti mini- mus manus	Little finger abduction

Note: Anatomic overlap is considerable and often bewildering; therefore, this table is not meant to be a strict anatomic delineation but rather a tool to localize root lesions.

muscles is particularly common but difficult to explain: C8-T1 roots innervate the intrinsic hand muscles, yet nerve root compression rarely affects that level. Similar so-called pseudoulnar signs can be seen with high cord compression, even as high as the level of foramen magnum. A commonly quoted explanation is that of venous back pressure with maximum venous dilatation or stagnation at C8-T1.

Fasciculations

Fasciculations are common and do not necessarily imply a progressive wasting disease of the anterior

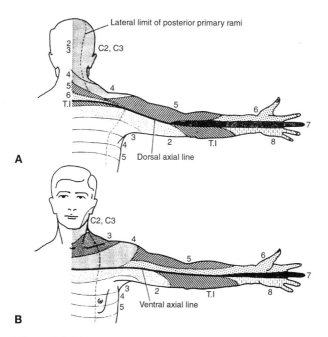

Figure 3-1. Diagram of the dermatomes in the upper limbs. **(A)** Posterior aspect. **(B)** Anterior aspect. Although there is variability and overlap across the interrupted lines, there is little or no overlap across the continuous lines (i.e., the ventral and dorsal axial lines). The examiner should routinely choose one spot in the "middle" of a dermatome and test at that point in all patients. C4 usually terminates at the point of the shoulder, T3 is almost always in the axilla, and T4 spreads across the chest so that C4 abuts T4 approximately at the nipple line. (Reprinted with permission from M Wilkinson. Cervical Spondylosis: Its Early Diagnosis and Treatment [2nd ed]. Philadelphia: Saunders, 1971;28.)

horn cells. Thus, in patients without sensory signs or symptoms but with weakness, wasting, fasciculations, and hyperreflexia, differentiation of spondylosis from motor neuron disease can be confusing, and the crucial finding in motor neuron disease is signs of denervation either clinically or on electromyographic testing in muscles remote from cervical myotomes.

Weakness

Because some muscles are stronger than others, evaluation of weakness requires a "gold standard" to be certain of the physical sign; a 300-lb football player is likely to find an 85-year-old woman "weak" in all muscle groups. If one can overcome the action of a muscle by resisting or opposing its action close to the joint that it moves using an equivalent equipotential muscle of the examiner, (e.g., fingers test fingers and the whole arm tests the biceps) that muscle is, by definition, weak. The examiner should then grade the weakness. A five-point grading system is usually used: 5 indicates normal muscle strength, 4 indicates that muscle weakness is present, 3 indicates that sufficient strength exists for the muscle to resist gravity, 2 indicates that the muscle is unable to move the joint against gravity, 1 indicates a flicker of movement about the joint, and 0 indicates complete paralysis. Varying degrees of

Table 3-2. Schema for grading weakness

Grade	Degree of weakness
0	Paralysis
1	Only a flicker on volition
2	Able to move a joint if gravity is eliminated
3	Able to move a limb against gravity
4*	Mild, moderate, or severe weakness, but more strength than grade 3
5	Normal

*Grade 4 is generally expanded, and every examiner should be familiar with his or her own interpretation of this expansion so that, on repeat examination, improvement or deterioration can be evaluated.

weakness exist within grade 4; therefore, it is common practice to expand grade 4 in some way. Provided the system used is constant and replicable by the examiner, any expansion will do. A good expansion is simply to add the adjectives "mild," "moderate," or "severe" to grade 4 (Table 3-2).

Having established the distribution and severity of weakness, the examiner should make an anatomic diagnosis from a consideration of the pattern of weakness. In cervical spondylosis, the pattern of weakness is almost always myotomal or radicular in the upper limbs, and weakness in the lower limbs is tract related—that is, upper motor neuron in distribution, discussed below.

Sensory Loss

Appreciation of pain sensation is tested with a new pin, but the patient should first be trained to recognize the difference between sharp and blunt. Decreased sensation for the pinprick often accompanies loss of thermal sensation, which is easily tested with a cold tuning fork. Light touch is tested with a wisp of cotton, vibration sense is tested by applying a tuning fork to a finger, and position sense is tested by stabilizing the proximal joints and altering the position of the most distal part of a finger. For the latter exercise, the patient's eyes should be closed.

If a deficit exists, it will likely be for pinprick appreciation. Again, the pattern of sensory loss allows for an anatomic diagnosis of the root involved, and the dermatomal map should be consulted. Loss of position sense in the fingers is rare in cervical spondylosis, which is usually maximal from C4 to C7; usually proprioceptive loss in the fingers with intact sensation in the toes suggests a very high cord lesion. A glove distribution of loss of pinprick and light touch is occasionally seen.

Reflex Change

Although one might expect reflex loss with an appropriate root lesion, reflex change in the upper limbs is extremely variable in cervical spondylosis. The biceps reflex is occasionally absent with a C5 root lesion, and, likewise, the triceps reflex is absent with a C6-C7 lesion. More commonly, however, hyperreflexia is present throughout. This may be explained by the presence of a mixed upper and lower motor neuron lesion. The finding is similar to that in motor neuron disease, again a situation with mixed upper and lower motor neuron pathophysiology. An absent biceps reflex with flexion of the fingers or even a brief contraction of the triceps on striking the biceps tendon at the elbow is referred to as an *inverted biceps jerk*. Although the reflex arc is nonfunctional, vibrations set up in adjacent muscles are sufficient to trigger local contractions. An inverted biceps jerk implies a C5 root lesion.

CORD SIGNS

Variability from patient to patient is the keynote of cervical spondylotic myelopathy. Cervical cord compression may result in any combination of motor or sensory long-tract signs as well as bladder dysfunction. The severity of the pathology on imaging studies often does not correlate with the physical signs found.

Spasticity

Spasticity or hypertonia in the lower limbs can result in a gait disorder. The legs are held adducted, the gait is narrow based, and the toes scrape audibly on the ground. On the examining couch, the feet are held fairly rigid on the legs when the legs are rotated briskly from side to side. Frank clasp-knife rigidity may be present at the knees, and clonus may be present at the ankles.

Weakness

Weakness in the lower limbs due to motor tract dysfunction conforms to the pattern of upper motor neuron dysfunction. The muscles that are particularly affected are the hip flexors, the foot and toe dorsiflexors, the hamstrings, and the thigh abductors. The other lower limb muscles may be normal in strength or, if weak, are relatively stronger than the muscles mentioned above.

Reflexes

Although hyperreflexia with increased knee and ankle tendon reflexes is usually present in myelopathy, the plantar responses may or may not be abnormal. Physiologically, an extensor plantar response indicates dysfunction in the pyramidal tract, whereas hypertonia and hyperreflexia are generated by extrapyramidal dysfunction—that is, dysfunction of nonpyramidal motor descending cord tracts. Although hypertonia and hyperreflexia are often seen hand-in-hand with extensor plantar responses, the absence of an extensor plantar response does not exclude myelopathy.

Sensory Loss

Cervical cord compression can result in sensory signs related to the ascending spinothalamic or posterior column tracts. In addition, clinicians should also consider sensory signs arising from dysfunction in the center of the cord. The spinothalamic and posterior column tract anatomy is likened to an onion peel arranged in somatotopic fashion. In the case of the spinothalamic tract, the peripheral part of the tract carries sensation from sacral dermatomes, and in orderly fashion from the outer part of the tract to the inner part, there follows foot, leg, trunk, and arm somatotopic areas. In the posterior columns, the more lateral part of the tract carries sensation from the arm, and the central part of the tract conveys sensation moved from the foot. Dysfunction, however, is not synonymous with pathology, and extrinsic compression of the cord can result in any combination of complete or partial tract dysfunction. Root signs give the clue to localization of the segmental level.

When the cervical cord is compressed, dysfunction can be patchy, progressive, or both. Thus, spinothalamic tract sensory loss for pinprick in the lower limbs or trunk can also be patchy and can mimic dermatomal loss. Furthermore, the level of the sensory loss can ascend gradually to approach the cervical dermatomes, or the reverse can hold with descending levels. It is only when a definite root sign is found by virtue of weakness, dermatomal loss, or a dropped reflex that a precise segmental level of dysfunction can be ascertained. If the dysfunction is mainly in the central cord, the peripheral cord areas are spared, resulting in normal sensation for pinprick in the sacral areas with loss in higher dermatomal areas—the phenomenon of *sacral sparing*.

Sometimes the only sensory tract loss is that relating to the posterior columns, resulting in loss of position sense, a positive Romberg sign, and sensory gait ataxia.

Cord compression can also result in central cord dysfunction. The clinical picture is that of dissociated sensory loss in the distribution of the cervical dermatomes—that is, loss of pinprick and temperature sensation with retention of light touch vibration sense and position sense. There may be no long-tract signs in the lower limbs. The bedside picture is similar to that found in syringomyelia.

FURTHER READING

Brain WR, Wilkinson M. Cervical Spondylosis and Other Disorders of the Cervical Spine. Philadelphia: Saunders, 1967.

Good DC, Couch JR, Wacasar L. "Numb clumsy hands" and high cervical spondylosis. Surg Neurol 1984;22:285.

Ronthal M. Weakness. In MA Samuels, S Feske (eds), Office Practice of Neurology. New York: Churchill Livingstone, 1996.

Sabin TD, Dawson D. Sensory Loss and Paresthesias. In MA Samuels, S Feske (eds), Office Practice of Neurology. New York: Churchill Livingstone, 1996.

Pathophysiology

The term *cervical spondylosis* is used to describe a degenerative disorder of the cervical spine characterized by disk degeneration with disk space narrowing, bone overgrowth producing spurs and ridges, and hypertrophy of the facet joints, all of which in turn compress cord or nerve root. Hypertrophy of the ligaments, particularly of the ligamentum flavum but also of the anterior longitudinal ligaments, is also present, and calcification may contribute to compression of neurologic structures. Hypertrophic osteophytes are present in approximately 30% of the population, and the incidence increases with age. The degree of bony change, however, does not correlate with the severity of the signs and symptoms that vary and fluctuate. The clinical course may be episodic or progressive, deterioration may be slow or rapid, or the patient may remain static for years.

The normal anatomy of the cord and its coverings is depicted in Figs. 4-1 and 4-2.

RADICULOPATHY

In radiculopathy, as opposed to myelopathy, the concept of compression or trauma to the root with appropriate signs and symptoms is easy to appreciate. Acute disk herniation is sometimes referred to as *soft-disk pathology*, as opposed to *hard-disk pathology*, which refers to chronic bony changes or spurring and ridging that are osteoarthritic reactions to wear and tear or previous trauma. Acute disk herniation is likely to produce signs and symptoms related to a single cervical root with severe brachialgia, myotomal weakness, dermatomal sensory loss, and loss of the appropriate tendon reflex. Conversely, osteophyte formation is usually multilevel, and although a crisp nerve root syndrome may be seen, multilevel involvement with multilevel signs and symptoms is often present.

In cervical spondylosis, compression of the nerve roots as they traverse the exit foramina cannot all be due to bone spurring; if that were the case, the signs and symptoms would not fluctuate, and the natural history of root dysfunction in cervical spondylosis would not be one of relapse and remission. There

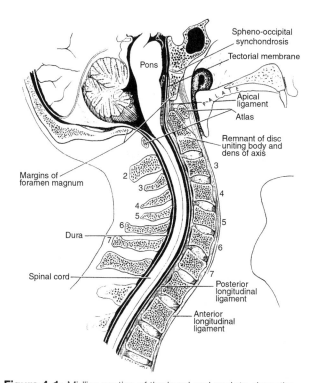

Figure 4-1. Midline section of the head and neck to show the relations of the dura, spinal cord, and hind brain to the bones, ligaments, and joints between the bodies of the vertebrae. Note the normal cervical lordosis, the relations of the anterior and posterior longitudinal ligaments to the intervertebral disk, and the ligaments at the cranio-vertebral junction. (Reprinted with permission from M Wilkinson. Cervical Spondylosis: Its Early Diagnosis and Treatment [2nd ed]. Philadelphia: Saunders, 1971;14.)

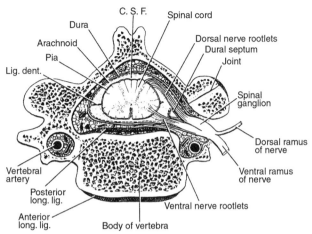

Figure 4-2. Relations of dura to bone and roots of nerve shown in an oblique transverse section. On the right, the relations between the emergent nerve and the synovial joint are seen, but the joint between the vertebral bodies is not in the plane of section. (C.S.F. = cerebrospinal fluid; Lig. dent. = ligamentum dentatum; long. lig. = longitudinal ligament.) (Reprinted with permission from M Wilkinson. Cervical Spondylosis: Its Early Diagnosis and Treatment [2nd ed]. Philadelphia: Saunders, 1971;18.)

must, therefore, be reversible soft-tissue pathology in the exit foramina, and it is usually regarded as inflammatory in origin. It is this soft-tissue reaction that responds to immobilization and allows for improvement, which occurs in 80–90% of patients treated appropriately. Fixed or persistent root signs suggest demyelination, scarring secondary to pressure, or both, and perhaps even axonal injury.

MYELOPATHY

An *acute* large-disk herniation can compress the spinal cord and result in a variety of long-tract signs below the level of compression. Extrinsic cord compression can cause dysfunction of any component of the cord at that level, and it is impossible to predict what combination of signs will be found below the level of compression. Root signs, however, are a hard pointer to the segmental level of pathology, and without them, no definite localization is possible.

The pathogenesis of myelopathy in *chronic* cervical spondylosis is a complex problem, and simple fixed mechanical cord compression cannot be the whole answer. Simple compression would neither allow for fluctuations nor account for the fact that decompression is not always curative.

Myelopathy is seen particularly in those individuals with a congenitally narrow spinal canal. Lateral radiographs allow for measurement of the posterior-anterior diameter of the canal (Fig. 4-3), and a diameter of less than 14–15 mm indicates a pre-existing narrow neural canal or spinal stenosis. The cord in spinal stenosis is vulnerable to compression by disk or

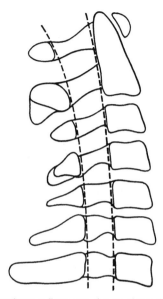

Figure 4-3. Continuous lines are drawn along the most anterior part of the spinous processes and along the most posterior part of the vertebral bodies. The anteroposterior diameter of the spinal canal at any level is determined by the distance between the two dotted lines. (Reprinted with permission from M Wilkinson. Cervical Spondylosis; Its Early Diagnosis and Treatment [2nd ed]. Philadelphia: Saunders, 1971;84.)

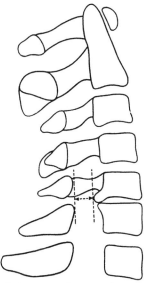

Figure 4-4. Osteophytes narrow the posterior-anterior diameter of the canal. (Reprinted with permission from M Wilkinson. Cervical Spondylosis: Its Early Diagnosis and Treatment [2nd ed]. Philadelphia: Saunders, 1971;86.)

osteophytes that further narrow the neural canal (Fig. 4-4). Spinal dimensions in patients with spondylotic myelopathy range from 7 to 17 mm. As osteophytic ridging develops anteriorly and hypertrophy of the ligamentum flavum develops posteriorly, the cord is pinched from both the front and rear, particularly in neck extension, which causes buckling of the ligament and aggravates the stenosis. Loose ligaments allow for subluxation in flexion and extension and aggravate the mechanical forces compressing the spinal cord. Massive osteophytes and ligamentous hypertrophy sometimes compress the cord even in the absence of congenital spinal stenosis.

The degree of cord compression seen on imaging studies does not necessarily correlate with the clinical signs of myelopathy. Relatively minor compression seen on magnetic resonance imaging may be the substrate of gait disorder and bladder dysfunction of some magnitude, and conversely, severe cord compression on magnetic resonance imaging may be clinically silent. Myelopathic signs fluctuate and even disappear in the absence of changes on the imaging studies. They may recur spontaneously, or deterioration may follow minor neck trauma. Patients with minor cord compression are at risk for clinical myelopathy in the event of neck injury, especially in automobile accidents when flexion/extension injuries are common, and when intubated for anesthesia for surgical procedures when hyperextension of the neck is favored by the anesthesiologist.

Because simple compression with or without local edema and demyelination cannot be the whole story, other explanations have been offered and are described in the remaining sections.

Vascular Compromise

Although no pathology in the anterior spinal artery has yet been demonstrated, surface, intramedullary, and radicular vessel insufficiency has been suggested, and blood flow in radicular vessels can be compromised by root fibrosis.

Intermittent Subluxation

Intermittent subluxation of vertebral bodies might cause intermittent cord compression with flexion/extension movements of the neck and yet remain undetected on sophisticated imaging studies, which produce only an image in the neutral position. Yet subluxation of a significant degree is present only in a minority of patients.

Traction of the Spinal Cord Against Osteophytes

In extreme flexion and extension movements, the spinal cord rides up or down in the spinal canal by as many as one or two segments. Furthermore, with flexion of the neck, the cord rides forward and impinges on the bony ridges of the spondylotic process. It has been postulated that friction of the cord on osteophytic spurs as it moves up and down may contribute to myelopathy (Figs. 4-5 and 4-6). This may explain why patients improve in a cervi-

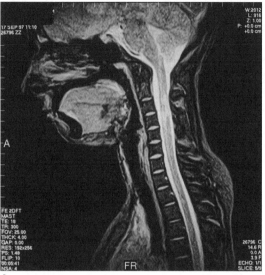

A

Figure 4-5. (A) Sagittal magnetic resonance image of the cervical spine of a patient with mild cervical spondylosis. This cut is made with the spine in neutral position. There appears to be ample room in the neural canal both posteriorly and anteriorly, so the cord is not touched. **(B)** The same patient is now scanned in neck flexion. The cord has moved to a relatively anterior position and is now in close apposition to anterior osteophytes. (Courtesy of Dr. Gerald O'Reilly; the treating neurologist was Dr. Charles Poser.)

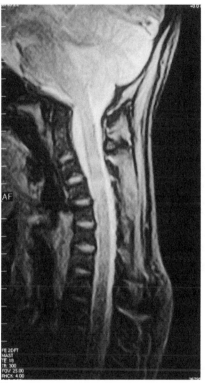

B

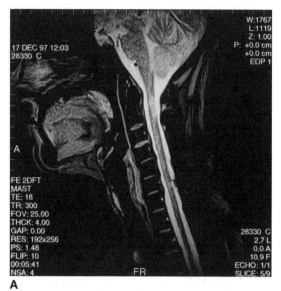

A

Figure 4-6. Another example of the cord bow-stringed anteriorly over moderate osteophytes in a patient with only mild cervical stenosis. **(A)** T1 sagittal image in the neutral position. **(B)** Same, but with flexion. The cord has moved anteriorly and is in close apposition to osteophytes. (During flexion and extension, the cord is free to move anteriorly and posteriorly and may be traumatized by anterior osteophytes on flexion. In extension, it may impinge on a thickened ligamentum flava.) (Courtesy of Dr. Gerald O'Reilly; the treating neurologist was Dr. Charles Poser.)

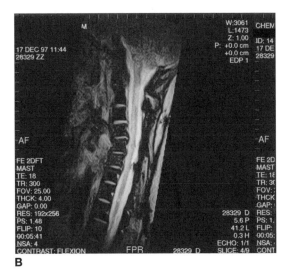

B

cal collar that restricts flexion/extension movements much more than rotation of the neck.

Insufficient Venous Return

In cervical cord compression at any segmental level and also in patients with foramen magnum space-occupying lesions, wasting and weakness with sensory loss in ulnar distribution is seen. Hand muscle wasting and weakness of the hands in spondylosis is frequent and suggests pathology at approximately C8-T1, yet the pathology is rarely seen at that particular level. A "pseudoulnar" sign is therefore regarded as false localizing. It has been suggested that compression interferes with venous return, which is upward, and that venous congestion and stagnant hypoxia maximal at C8-T1 cause the signs.

FURTHER READING

Adams CBT, Logue V. Studies in cervical spondylotic myelopathy. Brain 1971;94:557.

Adams CBT, Logue V. Studies in cervical spondylotic myelopathy. II. Movement and contour of the spine in relation to the neural complications of cervical spondylosis. Brain 1971;94:569.

Bohlman HH, Emery SE. The pathophysiology of cervical spondylosis and myelopathy. Spine 1988;13:843.

Breig A, Turnbull I, Hassler O. Effects of mechanical stresses on the spinal cord in cervical spondylosis: a study on fresh cadaver material. J Neurosurg 1966;25:45.

Gooding MR. Pathogenesis of myelopathy in cervical spondylosis. Lancet 1974;2:1180.

Gooding MR, Wilson CB, Hoff J. Experimental cervical myelopathy: effect of ischemia and compression of the canine cervical spinal cord. J Neurosurg 1975;43:9.

Hoff J, Nishimura M, Pitts L, et al. The role of ischemia in the pathogenesis of cervical spondylotic myelopathy:

a review and new micro-angiographic evidence. Spine 1977;2:100.

Juhl JH, Miller SM, Roberts GW. Roentgenographic variations in the normal cervical spine. Radiology 1962;78:591.

Nurick S. The natural history and the results of surgical treatment of the spinal cord disorder associated with cervical spondylosis. Brain 1972;95:101.

Medical Treatment

Because the exact pathophysiology of myelopathy and radiculopathy is not entirely clear, it is difficult to choose one form of treatment over another. No controlled trials of treatment for cervical spondylosis exist, nor does proof that any particular type of treatment is better than another or even better than the passage of time. A management plan that seems to work for most patients is offered in this chapter. The objective of medical treatment is to treat symptomatically and to minimize tissue damage. To this end, one can utilize both "mechanical" and drug therapy in treatment. Medications are offered if the response to simpler measures is unsatisfactory.

MECHANICAL TREATMENT

Neck Pain

Patients frequently complain of a stiff neck or muscle contraction headache on awakening in the morning. During sleep, the patient frequently changes position, tosses and turns, and may even have a nightmare, all resulting in excessive neck movement and irritation of pain-sensitive structures. Sleeping on two hard feather (not goose down, which is too soft) pillows is often very effective. Brand-name pillows in various shapes and compositions are expensive and usually no better than simple hard pillows. Local heat in the form of an electric warming pad applied to the back of the neck is both comforting and spasmolytic. Some physical therapists recommend ice packs.

If sleeping on hard pillows is ineffective, the patient should be instructed to sleep in a cervical collar. A soft foam collar is usually comfortable but, on occasion, cannot be tolerated and prevents sleeping. A hand towel rolled up to the width of a collar and secured around the neck with a safety pin may work just as well. As the symptoms subside, compliance decreases, but the collar should be saved for treatment of the next exacerbation. The collar should be used also on long automobile and airplane trips and when at the movies. Patients who spend a good deal of time peering at computer screens should use the collar at the computer.

Other simple home remedies include massage of the tense posterior cervical muscles with an electric hand vibrator and over-the-door cervical traction. A cervical contraction apparatus consists of a halter, a rope or cord, and a water container that has graduation marks to indicate the weight of the water in the container. The water bag should never be filled in excess of 5–7 lbs. The patient sits on one side of an open door with the halter on his or her head, and the cord passes over the door to the other side with the water bag hanging from its distal end. Ten- to 20-minute sessions are recommended, and some patients report benefit.

Physical therapy relieves muscle spasm and alleviates muscle contraction headache. The immediate benefit is short lived, and a course of treatment is often prolonged over many weeks. Despite the added cost, patient satisfaction is high. The physical therapist should be asked to apply heat, ultrasound, and massage. Neck manipulation should be avoided, and active exercise during a symptomatic period usually aggravates, rather than suppresses, symptoms. It is, in any case, difficult to understand what the benefit of neck exercise is.

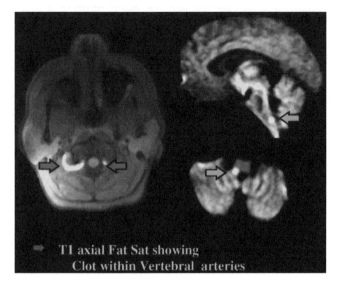

Figure 5-1. Magnetic resonance image of a patient who complained of vertigo immediately after chiropractic neck manipulation. The fat saturation image demonstrates a clot in the vertebral arteries secondary to dissection. The diffusion-weighted images in sagittal and axial planes show an infarction in the lateral medulla.

Chiropractic therapy is mentioned only to point out that manipulation of the cervical spine is dangerous (Fig. 5-1). Patients often report a significant effect in relieving pain—by an unknown mechanism—but the treatment has to be repeated fairly frequently. Approximately 12 million Americans undergo spinal manipulation therapy every year; the only published randomized controlled trial did not demonstrate that manipulation was significantly helpful. One review, however, described 138 cases with serious complications, including posterior circulation stroke and even death.

Root Pain

Root symptoms and signs respond partially or completely to immobilization with a cervical collar in 80–90% of patients. Initially, a soft collar is worn day and night for 2–3 weeks, and, thereafter, the patient is instructed to continue sleeping in the collar for another month or so. As with all cervical therapy, however, the use of cervical collars is controversial. Some therapists believe that a collar makes the neck weak. Because it is difficult to evaluate neck strength, the weakness hypothesis has been neither tested nor validated.

Myelopathic symptoms also frequently respond to neck immobilization with a collar. In many older patients who refuse surgery or for those patients who are unfit for surgery, immobilization is the treatment of choice. These patients use a collar on a daily basis as they would any other article of apparel and can be maintained pain free and without significant myelopathic symptoms for years.

Patients often ask, "What can I do or not do, and what should I avoid?" The golden rule is to avoid what hurts. "If it hurts, don't do it!"

DRUG TREATMENT

The foremost principle of drug treatment is to control pain, which may be accomplished by the use of analgesics, muscle relaxant drugs, and antidepressants. The following sections apply to both neck and root pain.

Analgesics

As with any form of pain-control therapy, one uses "what it takes" to render the patient pain free or almost so. Analgesics should be used in ascending order of strength until an effect is seen. Thus, the range is from simple aspirin or acetaminophen, to ibuprofen and other nonsteroidal anti-inflammatory drugs (NSAIDs), to propoxyphene in various combinations. If these medications produce no effect, tramadol and then codeine should be used. Very potent narcotics are rarely necessary, but they may be required in acute disk herniation with severe pain. The notion that NSAIDs treat an inflammatory disease of the neck is attractive but unproved and the benefit is likely produced mainly via their analgesic potential. The new

NSAIDs (cyclo-oxygenase 2 inhibitors) have not yet been used or evaluated for cervical spondylosis.

Antidepressants

The rationale for antidepressant use is partly because patients with chronic pain syndromes become depressed, but the tricyclics in particular have been shown to have an analgesic effect distinct from their effect on depression itself. Amitriptyline, 25–50 mg at night, is often a first choice, but many patients find the anticholinergic and sedative side effects disagreeable. Nortriptyline has fewer side effects. The analgesic response appears sooner (3–7 days) than the antidepressant effect (14–21 days). Tricyclics increase synaptic levels of dopamine, noradrenaline, and serotonin and may also bind to opiate receptors. The newer antidepressants, selective serotonin reuptake inhibitors, have almost no anticholinergic side effects and seem to work as well as traditional antidepressants, although the literature is controversial. Fluoxetine or sertraline, up to 50 mg per day, or, if night sedation is required, trazodone, 50 mg at night, are reasonable choices.

Muscle Relaxants

Diazepam, 2 mg three times a day, is the first-choice muscle relaxant. A number of specific designer muscle relaxants are on the market; cyclobenzaprine and methocarbamol are reasonable choices. None seem more effective than diazepam, and all are sedating in various degrees. Patients who show no response to a conservative course of treatment for 3–4 weeks should undergo further study. An x-ray of the cervical spine should be performed to confirm spondylosis and exclude gross bone erosion.

Steroids

In patients with acute soft-disk herniation, steroids are often very effective as a "quick-fix" remedy. A short burst of prednisone, 40–60 mg daily for a week, is unlikely to result in side effects and frequently relieves symptoms.

FURTHER READING

Cusick JF. Pathophysiology and treatment of cervical spondylotic myelopathy. Clin Neurosurg 1991;37:661.

David J, Modi S, Aluko AA, et al. Chronic neck pain: a comparison of acupuncture treatment and physical therapy. Br J Rheumatol 1988;37:1118.

Dillin W, Booth R, Cuckler J, et al. Cervical radiculopathy: a review. Spine 1986;11:988.

Harris PR. Cervical traction: review of literature and treatment guidelines. Phys Ther 1977;57:910.

Martin GM, Corbin KB. An evaluation of conservative treatment for patients with cervical disc syndrome. Arch Phys Med Rehabil 1954;35:87.

Powell FC, Hanigan WC, Olivero WC. A risk/benefit analysis of spinal manipulation therapy for relief of lumbar or cervical pain. Neurosurgery 1993;33:73.

Ronthal M, Rachlin JR. Cervical Spondylosis. In RT Johnson, JW Griffin (eds), Current Therapy in Neurologic Disease (5th ed). St. Louis: Mosby, 1997;76–79.

Swezey RC. Chronic neck pain. Rheum Dis Clin North Am 1996;22:411.

Tan JC, Nordin M. Role of physical therapy in the treatment of cervical disc disease. Orthop Clin North Am 1992;23:435.

Surgical Treatment

SURGERY

Although surgery for cervical spondylosis may be the most common neurosurgical procedure performed in the United States, its efficacy is still unproven. The literature is sparse, and not all surgeons agree even on the technical approach to the spondylotic neck.

In a 1992 review of the literature, Rowland reported that, of 261 patients subjected to posterior cervical laminectomy, 60% improved, 34% were unchanged, and 6% were worse. Of 385 patients surgically treated with an anterior approach, 52% were better, 24% were unchanged, and 23% were worse after the operation. Of 136 patients treated conservatively without surgery, 44% improved, 33% were unchanged, and 23% deteriorated. Moreover, the perioperative morbidity is generally in the range of 4–5%. No controlled trial of surgery versus conservative treatment has been reported, and the plan suggested is based on customary and usual management principles.

Surgery in cervical spondylosis is generally reserved for fit patients with myelopathy or for patients with acute disk herniation who do not respond to immobilization. If the pathogenesis of myelopathy is by way of cord compression, cord decompression is logical and reasonable. The goal of surgery is to decompress the spinal cord and affected nerve roots.

Surgical intervention is rarely beneficial in patients without clear-cut radiologic evidence of cord or root compression, regardless of the clinical presentation. Obtaining this evidence requires impeccable imaging, and the gold standard is magnetic resonance imaging. Occasionally, computed tomography is helpful in delineating calcification in the posterior longitudinal ligament. Why the operation is not uniformly successful must relate to our imperfect understanding of the precise pathogenesis of cervical spondylotic myelopathy.

Although Rowland's review of the literature is discouraging, other series suggest a better outcome with surgery in selected cases; one might expect that approximately 50% of patients return to full employment and that another 30–40% return to light employment 2–3 months after surgery. More aggressive surgeons believe that, with critical stenosis (canal diameter <8 mm)—even with minimal signs of myelopathy—decompression should be considered. Such patients are at risk of myelopathy from the point of view of natural history, and especially so if subject to trauma with a flexion/extension injury. Most practitioners follow a conservative course and consider surgery only if significant clinical myelopathy is present. Although a conservative plan requires careful observation, patients in this category can lead perfectly normal lives for many years. These patients should not engage in exercises that stress the neck, although many of them even ski, wearing a collar!

If surgery of any kind, not specifically cervical surgery, is undertaken, fiberoptic intubation while the patient is awake should always be used to minimize the risk of hyperextension injury to the cord.

The pain of acute radiculopathy due to a soft-disk herniation compressing a single nerve root and in which there is no response to immobilization and steroids is often dramatically cured by an anterior diskectomy. Foraminotomy is almost never performed today; almost all chronic radicular syndromes improve with time.

In the presence of myelopathy, if flexion/extension x-ray films of the cervical spine demonstrate instability, cervical fusion should be considered.

The exact approach, whether it is from the front with diskectomy and anterior cervical fusion or from the rear with laminectomy, should be the decision of the surgeon. It is difficult to prove the benefit of one approach over the other, but it seems reasonable that the direction of approach should be the direct and shortest route to the site of greatest cord compression.

Single-level anterior diskectomy and fusion yield reasonably good results, but after 5–10 years, the disk above or below the level of fusion, which has now been subject to extra stress, often degenerates, and further surgery may be required. After fusion, rigid neck braces are required for approximately 6–8 weeks until x-rays verify solid fusion.

If more than two levels are involved in the pathology, the surgeon should consider a multilevel posterior laminectomy, rather than a multilevel anterior fusion procedure that ultimately subjects the remaining disks to even more mechanical wear and tear. Decompression from the rear allows the cord to ride backward and avoid being compressed by the anterior ridging. Foraminotomy may be combined with laminectomy. Even fusion can be accomplished via a posterior approach, and the transverse processes can be wired or grafted with a rib graft. It is, however, impossible to remove ventrally placed osteophytes from the posterior approach.

COMPLICATIONS

Cord damage, possibly caused by careless technique or hyperextension during intubation, is a complication of surgery. With foraminal decompression, nerve root damage may occur, particularly at C5, but recovery can be expected in approximately 90% of patients. Recurrent laryngeal nerve injury, carotid artery trauma, failed fusion, or bone graft migration or instability are all rare complications of the anterior approach.

Poor outcomes were reviewed by Clifton: Fifty-six patients were studied, and the reasons for an unfavorable result included a wrong diagnosis (14.3%), spinal cord atrophy (26.8%), diffuse spinal stenosis (28.6%), and failure of decompression (57.1%). Failed surgery may therefore be due to a technical fault in as many as 85% of patients who have a bad result. For patients who are about to undergo surgery, the presence of a T2 white spot in the cord at the level of the compression is a poor prognostic factor.

More radical surgical treatment for multisegmental cervical spondylosis with vertebral body replacement, decompression, bone grafting, and osteosynthesis has been advocated. Time will tell.

FURTHER READING

Clifton AG, Stevens JM, Whitear P, Kendall BE. Identifiable causes for poor outcome in surgery for cervical spondylosis. Neuroradiology 1990;32:450.

Fairbank J. Trials and tribulations in cervical spondylosis [editorial]. Lancet 1998;352:1165.

Jeffreys RV. The surgical treatment of cervical myelopathy due to cervical spondylosis and disc degeneration. J Neurol Neurosurg Psychiatry 1986;49:353.

Rowland LP. Surgical treatment of cervical spondylotic myelopathy: time for a controlled trial. Neurology 1992;42:5.

Seifert V, Stolke D. Multisegmental cervical spondylosis: treatment by spondylectomy, microsurgical decompression, and osteosynthesis. Neurosurgery 1991;29:498.

Snow RB, Weiner H. Cervical laminectomy and foraminotomy as surgical treatment of cervical spondylosis: a follow-up study with analysis of failures. J Spinal Disord 1993;6:245; discussion, 250.

Symon L, Lavender P. The surgical treatment of cervical spondylotic myelopathy. Neurology 1967;17:117.

Prognosis of Cervical Spondylosis

Although cervical spondylosis is common, and cervical osteophytes are present in as many as 30% of the population, little correlation exists between the degree of anatomic abnormality and the clinical presentation. The correlation between spondylosis on x-ray or other imaging devices and clinical expression rises with age; it is rare to see an octogenarian who has a "normal" neck. Despite the high frequency of the condition, epidemiologic studies of the natural history and effects of treatment are sparse, and it is difficult to be certain about the prognosis.

The natural history of neck pain and muscle contraction headache has never been studied. In a related condition, soft-tissue injury of the neck, or so-called whiplash injury, in which the mechanism of pain is similar, approximately 40% of patients have persistent pain for at least 2 years, and sometimes longer with more severe injuries. In general, one fact is clear: the most likely outlook for symptomatic cervical spondylosis is a fluctuating course with recurrent episodes of pain, sometimes triggered by minor injury but often spontaneously reoccurring.

Cervical radiculopathy may be expected to follow a similar fluctuating course in terms of symptoms, but careful examination usually discloses minor radicular deficits even in asymptomatic individuals. The frequency of exacerbations and the result of treatment have never been prospectively or even retrospectively studied.

The only sign that is useful in predicting myelopathy is the presence or absence of a congenitally narrow spinal canal. Even exuberant osteophytes may not damage the cord in patients with a wide canal, and relatively mild osteophytes can cause indentation of the cord in patients with a narrow canal. In patients with myelopathy, the cord anterior-posterior diameter can be expected to range from 7 to 17 mm.

It is now generally accepted that surgical decompression is the treatment of choice in spondylotic myelopathy, but no recent studies have been reported, and no reported prospective controlled trials exist. Ten of 14 patients treated with a collar by Campbell and Phillips in 1960 improved. In 1963, Lees and Turner reported spontaneous improvement in six of 15 patients with "severe" disability followed for longer than 10 years. In 28 patients treated with a collar, 17 improved, seven were unchanged, and four worsened. Eighty-one patients with radicular symptoms never developed myelopathy at all. In a series reported by Nurick in 1972, 40% of 104 patients treated with a collar improved, 36% were unchanged, and 24% worsened. In 1967, Symon and Lavender found that 67% of patients had a steady progressive deterioration, and of 102 patients followed by Phillips in 1973, one-third who did not have an operation improved.

Rowland, in a 1992 review of the literature, reported the following figures: Of 261 patients subjected to cervical laminectomy, 60% improved, 34% were unchanged, and 6% worsened. Of 385 patients subjected to anterior surgery, 52% improved, 24% were unchanged, and 23% worsened. Of 136 patients treated conservatively, 44% improved, 33% were unchanged, and 23% worsened. One should also take into account perioperative morbidity. Again, perioperative morbidity varies from author to author, but, in general, 4–5% death or disability can be expected.

In 1990, Clifton and colleagues reviewed the cause for poor outcome in surgery for cervical spondylosis. Fifty-six patients were studied with the following results: Wrong diagnosis occurred in 14.3%, spinal cord atrophy in 26.8%, diffuse spinal stenosis in 28.6%, and failure of decompression in 57.1%. Failed surgery may therefore be due to a technical fault in as many as 85% of patients who have a bad result.

In the absence of hard data, all practitioners can do is bring experience into play. It seems that approximately 80% of patients with cervical myelopathy who have surgery either improve or, at the least, stop deteriorating.

Extraneous factors, such as pending litigation or psychiatric pathology, may often be crucial in the persistence of pain and alleged disability in patients with headache and mild radiculopathy. These individuals present an especially difficult diagnostic and therapeutic problem.

FURTHER READING

Adams CBT, Logue V. Studies in cervical spondylotic myelopathy. II. Movement and contour of the spine in relation to the neural complications of cervical spondylosis. Brain 1971;94:569.

Bernhardt M, Hynes RA, Blume HW, White AA. Current concepts review: cervical spondylotic myelopathy. J Bone Joint Surg Am 1993;75:119.

Campbell AMG, Phillips DG. Cervical disc lesions with neurological disorder. Differential diagnosis, treatment, and prognosis. BMJ 1960;2:481.

Clifton AG, Stevens JM, Whitear P, Kendall BE. Identifiable causes for poor outcome in surgery for cervical spondylosis. Neuroradiology 1990;32:450.

Lees F, Aldren Turner JW. Natural history and prognosis of cervical spondylosis. BMJ 1963;2:1607.

Nurick S. Natural history and results of surgical treatment of the spinal disorder associated with cervical spondylosis. Brain 1972;95:101.

Phillips DG. Surgical treatment of myelopathy with cervical spondylosis. J Neurol Neurosurg Psychiatry 1973;36:879.

Powell FC, Hanigan WC, Olivero WC. A risk/benefit analysis of spinal manipulation therapy for relief of lumbar or cervical pain. Neurosurgery 1993;33:73.

Rowland LP. Surgical treatment of cervical spondylotic myelopathy: time for a controlled trial. Neurology 1992;42:5.

Symon L, Lavender P. The surgical treatment of cervical spondylotic myelopathy. Neurology 1967;17:117.

Imaging

Regular x-rays are valuable for the following reasons:

- Degenerative changes are easily seen.
- Gross bone erosion is excluded.
- Lateral teleradiographs allow for accurate measurement of the posterior-anterior diameter of the neural canal.
- Flexion and extension views help to make the diagnosis of subluxation.

A posterior-anterior canal diameter of less than 15 mm indicates spinal stenosis.

Up to 3 mm of movement of one vertebra or the next (either above or below) on flexion or extension is considered to be within normal limits; more than 3 mm suggests an unstable cervical spine and is an indication for fusion in patients with myelopathy.

The advent of magnetic resonance imaging (MRI) has revolutionized the diagnosis of cervical spondylosis. Myelography is no longer necessary, and even computed tomographic scanning is now redundant and used only when MRI is not available or is contraindicated. Computed tomography may help also with the diagnosis of pathologic calcification—for example, in the anterior longitudinal ligament.

State-of-the-art MRI scanning is the procedure of choice when a surgical lesion is suspected, and the clinical indication for MRI scanning is the finding of myelopathic signs on examination. A lesser indication is failure of radicular signs and symptoms to resolve. Sagittal T1 and T2 and T2 axial images are routine. The sagittal T2 images tend to exaggerate the bony ridges and cord compression, and the T1 studies are more accurate in this regard. One should observe carefully for cord indentation on T1 images and for the extent of fluid both anterior and posterior to the cord to evaluate spinal stenosis.

Short case histories of patients with varying clinical presentations and the corresponding imaging studies are described.

An 84-year-old man complained of neck pain and stiffness that had responded to the use of a collar. He described a feeling of pressure on the top of his head. He had been involved in a motor vehicle collision 30 years previously when he was concussed. Neck movements were markedly limited; spasm and tenderness of the posterior cervical muscles were present. The straight x-ray showed well-marked spondylotic change with disk space narrowing and osteophytic spurring (Fig. 8-1). Encroachment on the intervertebral foramen was found at C5-C6.

A 63-year-old man presented to the neurology clinic for evaluation of familial action tremor. The examination revealed mild weakness of deltoid and biceps muscles as well as of hip flexion and toe extension bilaterally. This case was an example of incidentally discovered cervical spondylosis with myelopathy. The imaging demonstrated spinal stenosis with osteophytes indenting the spinal cord. The T2 images where the spinal fluid is "white" exaggerated the stenosis (Fig. 8-2). The axial images showed little spinal fluid around the cord (see Fig. 8-2).

A 75-year-old woman complained of staggering to the right. Her neck was spondylotic with restricted movement, but she was pain free. She had bilateral C5 weakness as well as wasting and weakness of the small muscles of the hands. The left triceps ten-

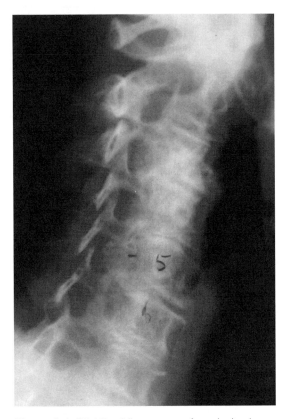

Figure 8-1. Slightly oblique x-ray of cervical spine showing multiple disk space narrowing and exuberant anterior and posterior osteophytes encroaching into the exit foramina of the cervical roots.

A

Figure 8-2. (A) Sagittal T1-weighted magnetic resonance image of the cervical spine. The cut is exactly in the midline, and although the neural canal is narrow, there appears to be space anterior to the cord. Nevertheless, osteophytes are present and indentations are seen in the anterior surface of the spinal cord.

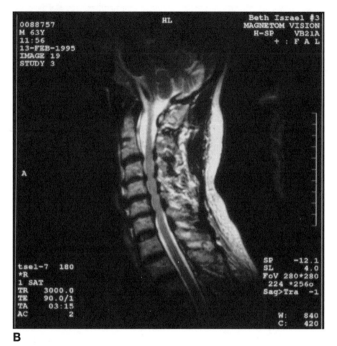

B

Figure 8-2. *Continued* **(B)** Sagittal T2-weighted magnetic resonance image of the cord. Although T2 images exaggerate the appearance of spinal stenosis, the neural canal is markedly narrow without space either in front of or behind the cord. **(C, D)** Axial T2-weighted images of the cervical spine at two levels demonstrating marked shortening of the anterior-posterior diameter of the neural canal produced by exuberant anterior osteophytes and also narrowing of the exit foramina, in part due to facet osteoarthritis on each side.

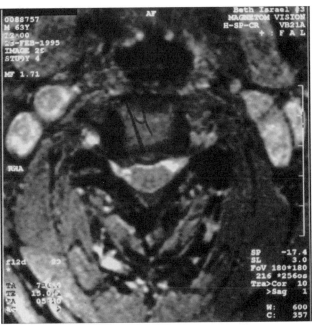

C

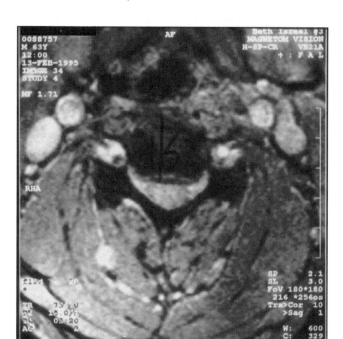

D

Figure 8-2. *Continued*

don reflex was absent. A mild paraparesis with flexor plantar responses was present. Use of a collar reversed her signs and symptoms, but 6 months after the initial visit, she was involved in a motor vehicle collision and returned with pain and stiffness in her neck and a well-marked paraparesis. She refused surgery, and use of a collar again reversed the physical signs. Over the next 6 years, she had recurrent episodes of paraparesis that were reversed by neck immobilization each time. Her case was an example of a fluctuating myelopathy responsive to immobilization. The MRI demonstrated mild spinal stenosis with some cord indentations (Fig. 8-3). It is likely that mild stenosis responds better to immobilization than severe stenosis with marked cord compression.

An 81-year-old female presented with "senile gait disorder" of multifactorial etiology. She had intermittent vertigo, cataracts, and a peripheral neuropathy with a stocking-pattern sensory loss of pinprick to midcalf bilaterally. She also had a moderate paraparesis and loss of position sense in the big toes, with a positive Romberg's sign. The MRI showed osteophytes at C4-C5 and C5-C6, with cord compression and some subluxation (Fig. 8-4). Her gait improved with the use of a collar.

A 63-year-old man complained of progressive difficulty using his hands for fine movements. He compensated with vision. He complained of urgency and

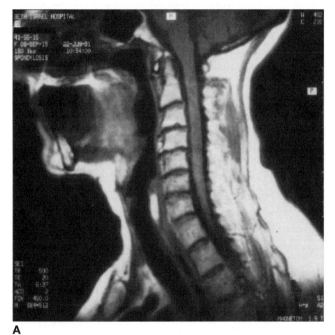

A

Figure 8-3. (A) Sagittal T1-weighted image of the cervical spine showing mild cervical stenosis. **(B)** Sagittal T2-weighted image of the cervical spine demonstrating osteophytic ridging touching the cervical cord.

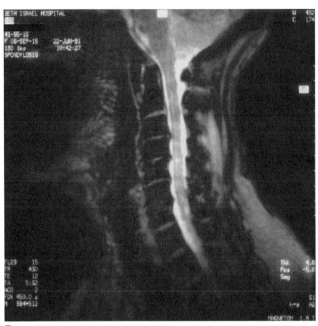

B

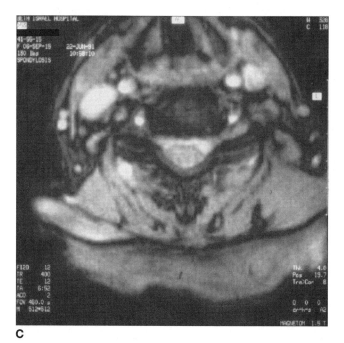

C

Figure 8-3. *Continued* **(C)** Axial T2-weighted image of the cervical spine showing exit foramen stenosis and mild neural canal stenosis. No cerebrospinal fluid shadow is present posterior to the cord.

A

Figure 8-4. (A) Sagittal T1-weighted image of the cervical spine showing narrowing of the disk spaces at C4-C5, C5-C6, and C6-C7 and with posterior osteophytes mainly at C4-C5, C5-C6 touching the spinal cord.

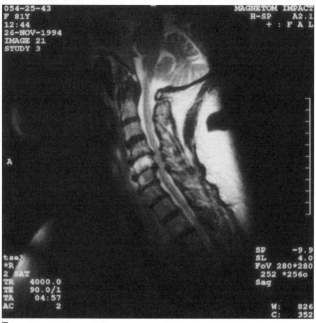

Figure 8-4. *Continued* **(B)** T2-weighted image demonstrating the osteophytes impinging on the cervical cord anteriorly, and also from the rear by hypertrophied ligamentum flava. **(C)** Axial T2-weighted image demonstrating marked reduction of the anterior-posterior diameter of the neural canal and narrowing of the exit foramina. There is no cerebrospinal fluid image either in front of or behind the cord, which is compressed and flattened.

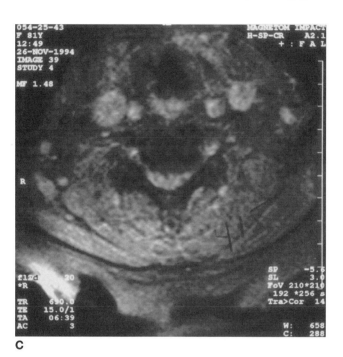

C

urgency incontinence. Atrophy with fasciculations in the shoulder girdle muscles and weakness of the hand intrinsics, finger extensors, wrist extensors, biceps, and deltoid bilaterally were present on examination. The upper limbs were areflexic. There was decreased pinprick sensation over C6-C7 dermatomes bilaterally. Proprioception was impaired in the fingers, and he had a mild paraparesis with flexor plantars and intact position sense. The MRI showed disk degeneration and subluxation at C4 on C5 and C6 on C7, with spinal stenosis at C4-C5 levels with cord compression (Fig. 8-5). Calcification of the anterior longitudinal ligament and foraminal narrowing were present.

A 78-year-old man had an anterior fusion and diskectomy at C4-C5 2 years before presentation. His hands improved, but his gait deteriorated, and he had urgency and urgency incontinence. He presented with a motor-only syndrome with fasciculations, wasting, and weakness in the upper limbs and a spastic paraparesis with extensor plantar responses. The MRI showed a wasted cord with multilevel compression and a large central osteophyte or calcified anterior longitudinal ligament, as well as the fusion (Fig. 8-6). A single-level diskectomy and fusion for

A
Figure 8-5. (A) T1-weighted sagittal image of the cervical spine showing a subluxation of C3 on C4 and C4 on C5 with degenerative bony change in the vertebral bodies at C5 and C6. The disk spaces are diffusely narrowed, posterior osteophytes are exuberant, the neural canal is encroached on, and the cord is deformed.

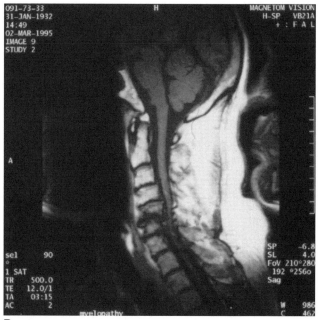

B

Figure 8-5. *Continued* **(B)** T1-weighted sagittal image off the midline showing wasting of the cord. The subluxation and degenerative bone disease is more apparent. **(C)** T2-weighted sagittal image demonstrating marked spinal stenosis, probable calcification in the posterior longitudinal ligament, and T2 shadows within the substance of the cord itself.

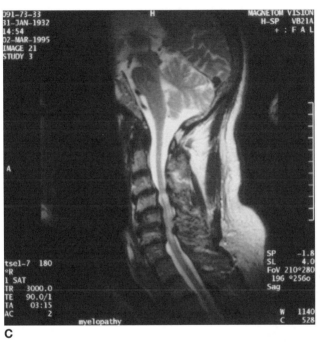

C

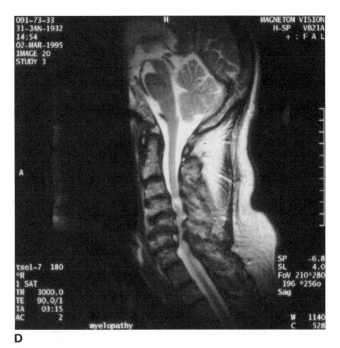

D

Figure 8-5. *Continued* **(D)** T2-weighted sagittal image off the midline demonstrating severe spinal stenosis that is due to anterior osteophytes and hypertrophy of the ligamentum flava or posteriorly.

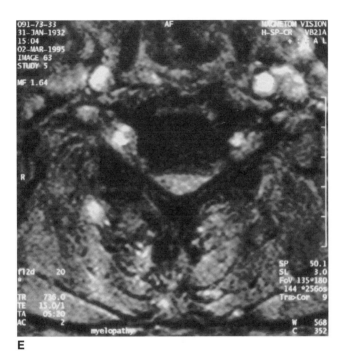

E

Figure 8-5. *Continued* **(E)** Axial T2-weighted image in the cervical spine demonstrating marked cervical stenosis due to a broad calcified ridge anteriorly. This is in part osteophyte, but calcification of the posterior longitudinal ligament may also be present. The spinal cord is markedly deformed with no space for spinal fluid either in front of or behind it. The exit foramina are markedly narrowed.

multilevel compression was the wrong operation and did not decompress the cord adequately. The patient subsequently had further surgery with multilevel decompression via a posterior approach and improved only marginally.

A 73-year-old woman presented with a gait disorder and had her hydrocephalus shunted. She did not improve. She complained of a bandlike feeling of tightness around the trunk and incontinence with loss of perineal sensation, and she had a 500-ml postvoiding residual volume of urine. Her mental status examination was normal, and she had a wasting and weakness of the hand muscles, spastic legs with extensor plantar responses, and a suspended level for pinprick, light touch, and temperature from T6 to Ll. The MRI showed "goose-neck" deformity and multilevel stenosis (Fig. 8-7).

Four years before an automobile collision, this 45-year-old woman had a positive Lhermitte's sign. After the collision, she developed C5 weakness and areflexia in the upper limbs and 1 year later had a mild paraparesis with extensor plantar responses. The MRI showed a disk prolapse at C5-C6 with cord compression but also a T2 hyperintensity opposite the body of

A

Figure 8-6. (A) T1-weighted sagittal image of the cervical spine demonstrating fusion of C4 and C5 but with subluxation of C3 on C4, osteophytes at that level, and a deformity of the cord at the same level.

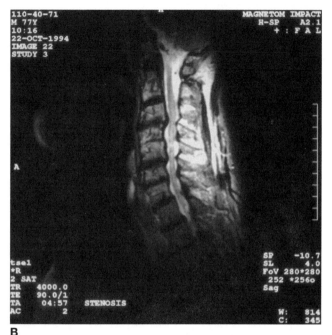

B

Figure 8-6. *Continued* **(B)** T2-weighted sagittal image of the cervical spine. Fusion at C4 and C5 is apparent. The disks are all desiccated; their shadows are dark on this image. There is sub-luxation of C3 on C4. Ridges at C3-C4 and C5-C6 encroach on the neural canal, and there is also some stenosis at C6-C7.
(C) Axial T2 image demonstrates a large central calcified posterior longitudinal ligament encroaching into the neural canal.

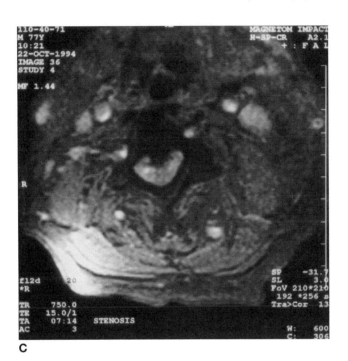

C

C6 (Fig. 8-8A). The cerebrospinal fluid was normal.
Because the T2 shadow was opposite the vertebral
body and not at the disk space, it was thought to represent demyelination (Fig. 8-8B, C). A brain MRI
showed numerous plaques in the white matter.

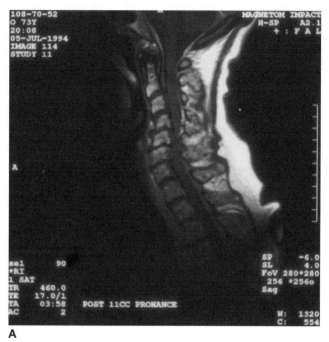

A

Figure 8-7. (A) Sagittal T1 image with narrowing of disk spaces at multiple levels, "goose-neck" deformity and marked spinal stenosis from C4 to C6. **(B)** Sagittal T2 image showing multiple cord indentations at the level of the spinal stenosis.

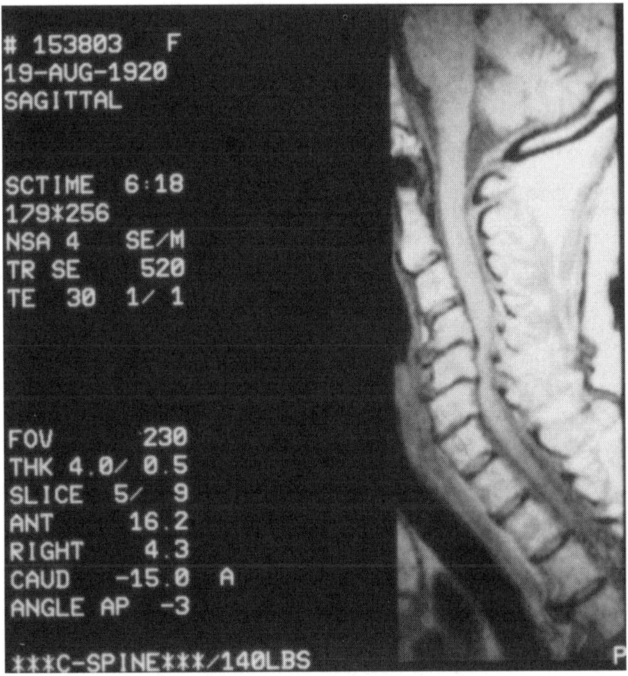

153803   F
19-AUG-1920
SAGITTAL

SCTIME   6:18
179*256
NSA 4   SE/M
TR SE   520
TE 30   1/ 1

FOV   230
THK 4.0/ 0.5
SLICE   5/ 9
ANT   16.2
RIGHT   4.3
CAUD   -15.0   A
ANGLE AP   -3

C-SPINE/140LBS

B

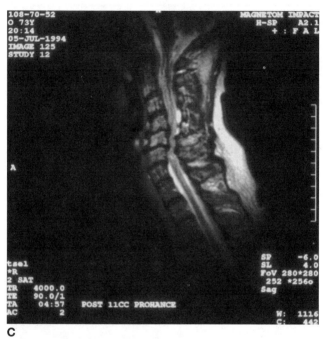

C

Figure 8-7. *Continued* **(C)** Sagittal T2 image just off the midline shows severe stenosis with cord compression from the rear by ligamentum flava and anteriorly by osteophytes. **(D)** Axial T2 image demonstrates marked spinal stenosis with reduction of the anteroposterior diameter of the neural canal and cord compression. There is no cerebrospinal fluid anterior or posterior to the cord, which is flattened. The exit foramina are relatively well preserved and open.

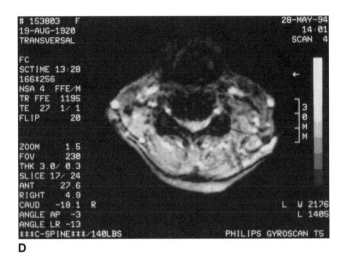

D

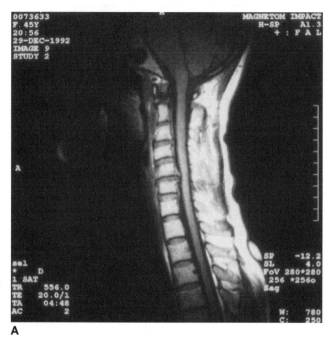

Figure 8-8. (A) Sagittal T1 projection showing disk prolapse at C5-C6 with cord indentation. There is also mild disk protrusion at C3-C4. **(B)** Sagittal T2 image that exaggerates the appearance of the disk protrusions at C3-C4 and C5-C6. There is a spot of T2 brightness in the cord adjacent to the body of C6.

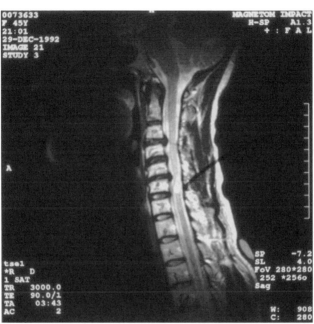

B

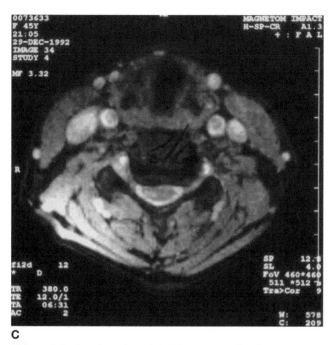

Figure 8-8. *Continued* **(C)** Axial T2 image at C5-C6 showing the disk prolapse anteriorly with flattening of the cord.

Differential Diagnosis of Cervical Spondylosis

Although cervical spondylosis is the most common neck problem seen in clinical practice, one should keep in mind that other pathologies can also produce cord and root signs and symptoms. A convenient way of approaching the problem is to divide the pathology into "medical" and "surgical" groups. Patients in the surgical group are amenable to invasive surgical therapy, whereas patients in the medical group are treated conservatively.

MEDICAL PATHOLOGY

Included under the medical pathology rubric are inflammatory and infective processes such as myelitis, which could be primarily demyelinating and part of

97

multiple sclerosis or a postinfectious radiculomyelitis. For the diagnosis of multiple sclerosis, a history of lesions separated in time and space is necessary. Multiple sclerosis may coesixt with cervical spondylosis, as can any other pathology. A single episode of myelitis could be the first attack of multiple sclerosis or may represent a postinfectious inflammatory episode. Here, often, but not always, a history of infection is present 2 or 3 weeks before the myelitis, but the nature of the primary infectious process is frequently obscure. A screen for antibodies to known infective agents may give the answer, and *Mycoplasma* should not be forgotten.

Herpes zoster myelitis is a good example of a primary viral infection of the cord and roots that is easily diagnosed because of the skin rash, but the cause of the radiculopathic pain may not be apparent before the rash appears. Human immunodeficiency virus can cause a chronic progressive vacuolar myelopathy; it usually occurs in the thoracic cord.

Granulomatous disease occasionally affects the cord or roots, and sarcoidosis, as well as infectious processes such as tuberculosis, should be considered. Tertiary syphilis is mentioned for historical value; pachymeningitis cervicalis presents with severe brachialgia and myelopathy, but cord infarction as part of meningovascular disease is still occasionally seen.

Cervical spondylosis sometimes presents with a motor-only syndrome, and approximately 5% of patients with the original diagnosis of cervical spondylosis with myelopathy have motor neuron disease. The electromyographic finding of widespread denervation, particularly in bulbar muscles, confirms the diagnosis.

Of the metabolic myelopathies, subacute combined degeneration is important because it is potentially treatable and presents with sensory symptoms in the hands with a posterior and lateral column dysfunction in the cord. Adrenoleukodystrophy often has a myelopathic component and represents another metabolic myelopathy.

Systemic or primary central nervous system vasculitis occasionally affects the cervical cord, and a microvascular angioma can present as a progressive myelopathy.

SURGICAL PATHOLOGY

Surgical disease in the cervical spine may cause cord compression from without—that is, extramedullary cord compression, root compression, or both, or may arise within the substance of the cord itself, an intramedullary process.

Nonspondylotic extramedullary root and cord compression is the major differential. Extramedullary cord compression may be caused by benign tumors, such as meningioma or neurofibroma, or by metastatic cancer. The primary tumors may cause bony change by way of scalloping of normal bone or enlarging the exit foramina, whereas metastatic disease erodes bone and grows in the epidural space and bone, sparing the disk. The cervical spine is the site of metastatic deposits in 15% of all patients with epidural metastases, and the most common primary tumors are in the lung or breast.

Bacterial infections usually settle in the disk, destroy it, and subsequently spread to the epidural space and bone, so that in patients with bone erosion, preservation of the disk space suggests a neoplastic process, whereas destruction of the disk indicates an infective pathology.

The dilatated veins of large dural vascular anomalies can compress the cord, and posterior fossa vascular anomalies occasionally cause high cervical cord edema because of venous back pressure.

Notwithstanding the fact that the most common cause of central cord dysfunction is extrinsic cord compression, primary intramedullary processes present with the identical clinical syndrome of dissociated sensory loss in cape distribution. The first thought is always of syringomyelia with or without a Chiari malformation, but a primary intramedullary cord glioma is always possible. Central nervous system lymphoma either isolated to the nervous system or part of a multiorgan process is becoming more common, and intramedullary metastatic deposits, usually from the lung, are seen occasionally.

After acute flexion/extension injuries, the pathology may be intramedullary hematoma (hematomyelia) rather than compression by disk.

Intramedullary abscess is extremely rare but devastating.

Because cervical spondylosis is so common, it often coexists with any of the above pathologies. The differential diagnosis is, in almost all cases, made on the basis of magnetic resonance imaging, spinal fluid, and blood studies. Biopsy may be required.

FURTHER READING

Brain WR, Wilkinson M. The association of cervical spondylosis and disseminated sclerosis. Brain 1957;80:456.

Burgerman R, Rigamonti D, Randle JM, et al. The association of cervical spondylosis and multiple sclerosis. Surg Neurol 1992;38:265.

Byrne TN, Waxman SG. Spinal Cord Compression: Diagnosis and Principles of Management. Philadelphia: FA Davis, 1990;9.

Whiplash Injuries

DEFINITION

The issues of whiplash injuries and whiplash-associated disorders (WADs) were reviewed and reported as a scientific monograph of the Quebec Task Force on Whiplash-Associated Disorders. According to that monograph, "Whiplash is an acceleration-deceleration mechanism of energy transfer to the neck. It may result from rear-end or side-impact motor vehicle collisions but can also occur during diving or other mishaps. The impact may result in bony or soft tissue injuries (whiplash injury), which in turn may lead to a variety of clinical manifestations (whiplash-associated disorders)." Although much has been written about WAD, the task force found only 346 papers of scientific merit in a review of more than 10,000 publications.

Rear-end motor vehicle collisions are responsible for approximately 85% of all whiplash injuries, and it is estimated that 1 million such injuries occur in the United States every year. The incidence varies by state and country, ranging from 13 to 106 per 100,000 inhabitants, and the syndrome is more common in females. Wearing a seatbelt, although not to be discouraged, may be a risk factor for whiplash. Most automobile headrests are ineffective because of poor design or improper positioning. A properly positioned headrest should be located so that the horizontal distance to the head is as small as comfortably possible, and the top edge should extend approximately 70 mm above the passenger's eye level.

A sudden hyperextension followed by hyperflexion of the cervical spine results in a so-called soft-tissue injury of the neck. Severe injuries may cause rupture of the anterior longitudinal ligament, horizontal avulsion of the vertebral end plates, occult fractures of the end plate, acute cervical disk herniation, focal muscular injury, and posterior interspinous ligament injury. Injury to the zygapophyseal joints, especially at C2-C3, has been suggested as the most common cause for chronic neck pain after whiplash.

The severity of the injury can be graded according to the following chart, and initial lesion severity predicts the persistence of symptoms:

Grade I: Neck complaints of pain, stiffness, or tenderness only, and no physical signs.

Grade II: Neck complaints together with physical signs consisting of decreased range of movement and point tenderness.

Grade III: Neck complaints together with neurologic signs: weakness, sensory loss, or absent reflex.

The presence of neurologic signs indicates a root injury due to either a disk protrusion or stretch injury. It is appropriate to segregate these patients from the more common soft-tissue injuries of the neck that carry a better prognosis. The advent of magnetic resonance imaging muddied the water, because disk protrusions may be seen in the absence of root signs, but no study has reviewed the prognosis of patients with disk rupture diagnosed only by magnetic resonance imaging.

The onset of neck pain occurs within 6 hours of the collision in approximately two-thirds of patients, within 24 hours in approximately one-fourth of patients, and within 72 hours in all other patients. A short latency to symptom onset is indicative of more severe neck trauma. Headache is a typical muscle contraction–type syndrome that is present in approximately 80% of patients 1 month after the injury. Other symptoms include dizziness, paresthesia, and cognitive and psychological symptoms. Dizziness is a nonspecific complaint, and the treating physician should inquire about the exact symptom. Patients with posterior cervical spasm frequently complain of mild imbalance, but true rotary vertigo usually implies a vestibular disturbance.

The prognosis is variable: In one representative series, the prognosis for persistent neck pain 6 or more months after the injury was as follows: grade I, 44%; grade II, 81%; and grade III, 90%. For headache, the prognosis was 37% for grade I, 37% for grade II, and 70% for grade III. Two years after the injury, neck pain was reported in 29–44% of patients.

In another series, neck pain was present in 74% of patients 10 years after the collision, although, in general, approximately 40% of patients report complete recovery at 2 years, and approximately 45% continue to have major complaints at 2 years after the collision.

Although it has been suggested that radiological features such as lack of cervical lordosis due to spasm or angulation of the neck suggest a poor prognosis, this is unproven. Pre-existing osteoarthritis predicts symptom persistence at 3 months, but not later.

The cause of persistent symptoms in patients with minor injuries is unknown. Little evidence exists for a structural basis for chronic whiplash in these patients.

Fifteen percent to 20% of patients complain of cognitive symptoms after whiplash (or concussion). In 1998, Alexander addressed the issue of brain damage and cognitive loss after whiplash, and his conclusions are briefly summarized: In primates, a pure deceleration force can produce diffuse axonal injury, the severity of which parallels the severity of the head injury as measured by the duration of coma, neurologic signs, and outcome. No credible evidence exists for this type of injury in humans who do not report loss of consciousness. There have been numerous reports of abnormal single photon emission computed tomography scans in patients complaining of cognitive loss after whiplash. The most common finding is decreased perfusion in frontal and anterior temporal regions, but similar findings are present in depression and anxiety disorders. It may be that the severity of pain triggers cognitive and vegetative symptoms. Instead of a *psychosomatic* illness, patients develop a *somatopsychic* illness. Severe secondary psychogenesis might account for the fact that patients with mild traumatic brain injury often report greater cognitive difficulty than severely injured patients after their early anosognosia has cleared. Single photon emission computed tomography cannot answer the question of causation and should not be regarded as a definitive test of brain damage for clinical or legal purposes or even as an appropriate clinical tool in the management of whiplash.

Although believed to be a significant factor by many neurologists, the influence of compensation and legal action in WAD is controversial. The dividing line between a relatively trivial injury and one of more significance should be drawn on the basis of the presence of neurologic signs. The lack of focal signs that suggest root or cord damage suggests that the injury is minor and of good prognosis, whereas the presence of such signs suggests a more severe injury and a worse prognosis.

Two studies of whiplash injuries in Lithuania, one retrospective and one prospective, merit closer consideration. Both showed a far lower incidence of neck pain and headache than contemporary Western reviews. In the prospective review, 210 subjects who had experienced rear-end collisions were matched to noninjured controls and interviewed by mailed questionnaires. The subjects probably all fell into grade I or II categories. Initial pain was reported by 47% of collision victims: 10% had neck pain alone, 18% had neck pain with headache, and 19% had headache alone. The median duration of the initial neck pain was 3 days, and maximum duration was 17 days. The median duration of headache was 4.5 hours, and the maximum duration was 20 days. At 1 year, no significant differences existed between the collision and control groups. In Lithuania, only a minority of car drivers are insured for personal injury. There is no expectation of the presence of symptoms or disability, and the therapeutic community is seldom involved. The inference from this study is that the expectation of disability and compensation may well be a significant factor in persistent WAD.

In patients with cognitive complaints without significant head injury, malingering may be more frequent, particularly in the context of litigation, but it is difficult to prove. The Amsterdam Short-Term Memory test measures underperformance. Underperformance may be due to malingering, an unconscious need for recognition in the face of medical skepticism, or even self-deception. Using this screen, underperformance in the context of litigation is twice as frequent in patients involved in litigation compared with symptomatic patients who do not have lawsuits pending.

A reasonable approach would be to separate WAD patients who have physical signs that suggest root or cord injury from those without root or cord injury signs: The former should be considered to have had a significant injury with an accordingly poorer prognosis. Similarly, in patients complaining of cognitive deficits, it is the severity of the head injury as measured by loss of consciousness that should determine the prognosis and organic validity of the symptoms—loss of consciousness or concussion implies a head injury with possible neuraxonal damage and not just whiplash.

The Quebec Task Force emphasizes that whiplash is essentially a benign condition with the majority of patients recovering, but it is the refractory minority that accounts for an inordinate proportion of the costs.

MANAGEMENT

Grade I patients who are alert—not obtunded by drugs or alcohol—do not require a radiologic study; all others should have x-rays performed. The finding of root or long-tract signs requires imaging.

If we are to practice evidence-based treatment, no foundation exists for the use of collars, rest, comma manipulation, mobilization, exercise, traction, postural alignment, spray and stretch treatment, transcutaneous nerve stimulation, electrical stimulation, ultrasound, laser, short-wave therapy, diathermy, heat, ice, massage, injections, muscle relaxants, and acupuncture.

What, then, can physicians offer? Practitioners vary in their approach. Because most cases of isolated WAD are self-limiting, reassurance, promotion of activity, and symptomatic therapy for pain are reasonable. Many patients report benefit from the use of muscle relaxants, hard pillows, sleeping in a collar, and antidepressants as analgesics. Gentle physical therapy helps to treat muscle spasm and also provides psychological support. Persistence of symptoms beyond 6 weeks may indicate more specialized advice, a multidisciplinary team evaluation, or both.

FURTHER READING

Alexander MP. In the pursuit of proof of brain damage after whiplash injury. Neurology 1998;51:336.

Norris SH, Watt I. The prognosis of neck injuries resulting from rear-end vehicle collisions. J Bone Joint Surg Br 1983;65:608.

Obelieniene D, Schrader H, Bovim G, et al. Pain after whiplash: a prospective controlled inception cohort study. J Neurol Neurosurg Psychiatry 1999;66:279.

Pearce JMS. Polemics of chronic whiplash injury. Neurology 1994;44:1993.

Radanov BP, Sturzenegger M, Di Stefano MA. Long-term outlook after whiplash injury. A 2-year follow-up considering features of injury mechanism and somatic, radiologic, and psychosocial features. Medicine (Baltimore) 1995;74:281.

Schagen S, Schmand B, de Sterke S, et al. Amsterdam Short-Term Memory test. A new procedure for the detection of feigned memory deficits. J Clin Exp Neuropsychol 1997;19:43.

Schmand B, Lindeboom J, Schagen S, et al. Cognitive complaints in patients after whiplash injury: the impact of malingering. J Neurol Neurosurg Psychiatry 1998;64:339.

Schrader H, Obelieniene D, Bovim G, et al. Natural evolution of late whiplash syndrome outside the medicolegal context. Lancet 1996;347:1207.

Spitzer WO, Skovron ML, Salmi LR, et al. Scientific monograph of the Quebec Task Force on Whiplash-Associated Disorders: redefining "whiplash" and its management. Spine 1995;20:8S.

Stovner LJ. The nosological status of the whiplash syndrome: a critical review based on a methodological approach. Spine 1996;21:2735.

Electromyography and Nerve Conduction Studies

Electrophysiologic testing is not indicated in every patient with neck pain, brachialgia, or both, but nerve conduction studies are useful to confirm or deny focal nerve pathology when the physical examination is equivocal and to define peripheral lesions, such as entrapment neuropathies complicating cervical pathology. Electromyography (EMG) demonstrates the anatomic distribution of partially denervated and healing muscle that, coupled with our knowledge of the normal anatomy, allows for localization of root, plexus, and nerve lesions. The studies are therefore indicated for patients suspected of having a complicating peripheral entrapment syndrome or when the diagnosis of root dysfunction is in doubt.

ELECTROMYOGRAPHY

A concentric needle electrode is inserted into the muscle to be studied, and the electrical activity generated by the muscle is displayed on an oscilloscope screen. At rest, normal muscle is silent. The patient is then requested to activate the muscle, gradually increasing the force of contraction. Single motor units are seen initially (Fig. 11-1), and more units are gradually recruited (Fig. 11-2) until the baseline is replaced by a continuous stream of electrical activity and cannot be seen—a full or complete interference pattern (Fig. 11-3).

The characteristics of normal motor units depend on the muscle studied, but for general somatic muscles, amplitude and duration as well as the number of positive and negative phases are measured. Thus, normal units have two to four phases (in limb muscles, approximately 12% may have five or more phases and are described as *polyphasic*), a duration of 2–15 ms, and an amplitude of 200 μv to 3 mv.

The following parameters are usually found in a typical EMG report and are therefore reviewed.

Insertional Activity

As the needle is inserted, a short burst of electrical activity occurs. Insertional activity is prolonged in

Right FDI

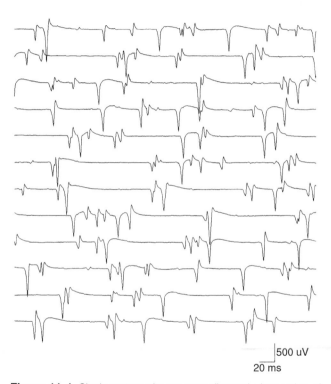

500 uV
20 ms

Figure 11-1. Single motor units are seen discretely. Inspection of the waveforms reveal that units of the same shape recur episodically. These are normal units—that is, not polyphasic. (FDI = first digital interosseus.) (Courtesy of Seward Rutkove, M.D.)

Right FDI

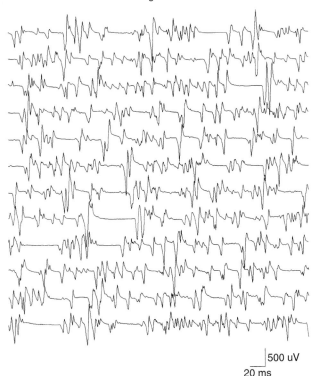

500 uV
20 ms

Figure 11-2. With greater volitional effort, more units have been recruited and, although possible, it is now difficult to pick out recurring units of the same shape. (FDI = first digital interosseus.) (Courtesy of Seward Rutkove, M.D.)

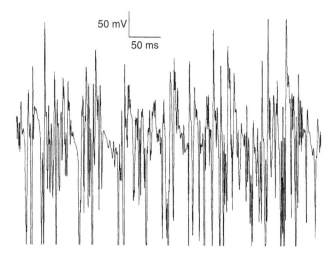

Figure 11-3. So many units have been recruited that it is difficult to make out the baseline. This is a full or normal interference pattern. (Courtesy of Seward Rutkove, M.D.)

denervated muscle, polymyositis, myotonia, and some other myopathies.

Activity at Rest

Fibrillation potentials are action potentials arising spontaneously from single muscle fibers at rest. They are low-voltage (20–300 μv), short-duration

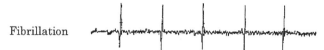

Fibrillation

Figure 11-4. Biphasic low-voltage potentials at rest indicating denervated or isolated myofibrils discharging spontaneously are called *fibrillations*. (Courtesy of Seward Rutkove, M.D.)

(<5 ms), and bi- or triphasic potentials. They recur at a firing rate of 2–20 per second and, over the speaker of the EMG machine, have a high-pitched, repetitive, clicking sound. They indicate denervation and appear 2–3 weeks after an acute neuropathic lesion. They are also seen in polymyositis and some other myopathies (Fig. 11-4).

Positive sharp waves are usually seen with fibrillation potentials and have approximately the same amplitude. There is an initial positive deflection followed by a slow negative recovery that can extend into a small negative wave. Positive sharp waves have the same significance as fibrillations, being present in acutely denervated muscle and in myopathies (Fig. 11-5).

Fasciculation potentials are produced by motor units that fire spontaneously and are similar to normal motor units in dimension. They produce irregular, dull, thumping sounds on the loudspeaker. Although they are occasionally seen in patients without pathology, they are usually seen in the presence of chronic

Positive Sharp
Wave

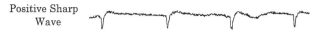

Figure 11-5. Positive sharp waves. (Courtesy of Seward Rutkove, M.D.)

partial denervation, particularly when the pathology is at the level of the anterior spinal horn cell.

Myotonic discharges are high-frequency trains of repetitive action potentials evoked by electrode movement, muscle percussion, or contraction with a waning and waxing amplitude and frequency that eventually settle spontaneously. On the speaker, they produce a sound likened to that of a motorcycle or dive-bomber. They are found mainly in myotonic disorders, occasionally in other myopathies, and rarely in neurogenic weakness.

Complex repetitive discharges (also called *pseudomyotonic discharges* or *bizarre high-frequency potentials*) have an abrupt onset and termination, and their amplitude and frequency remain constant. They are caused by direct cell-to-cell muscle fiber excitation occurring recurrently. They are seen in both chronic nerve and muscle disease.

Electrical Activity Seen with Volitional Contraction

Motor units are first observed with minimal muscle contraction to study individual units and then with maximal contraction to study the recruitment pattern.

In neuropathic disorders, functional motor units are reduced, and denervated muscle fibers are reinnervated by collateral branches sprouting from distal nerve fibers of surviving units. The collaterals spread over a wider area, and more time is taken to reach the relevant end plates. Conduction velocity in new collaterals is reduced. The net effect is to increase the duration of the potentials. Because the resultant functional motor unit has more muscle fibers, the unit is of large amplitude and is also polyphasic, each phase representing further myo-fibrils. In chronic active denervating diseases, such as motor neuron disease, the amplitude of the abnormal units may be as large as 5–10 mv and are called *giant potentials.*

As motor units drop out due to a neurogenic process, the density of electrical activity is reduced, and on maximal volition the baseline is not fully covered. When denervation is severe, it may be possible to recognize individual motor units firing very rapidly. The interference or recruitment pattern is reported as being reduced.

The EMG signs of denervation in the acute phase are fibrillation potentials; positive sharp waves and then later on fasciculations may be seen at rest. With reinnervation, on volitional long-duration,

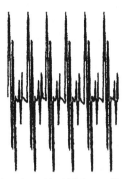

Figure 11-6. A reduced but high-amplitude recruitment pattern indicative of reinnervation. (Courtesy of Seward Rutkove, M.D.)

high-amplitude polyphasic motor units with a reduced recruitment pattern (Fig. 11-6) are seen. A neuropathic EMG in the cervical paraspinal muscles indicates radiculopathy in that the first branch after the root leaves the intervertebral foramen is to the cervical paraspinal muscles.

In myopathy, dissolution and fragmentation of individual muscle fibers are present. This results in low-amplitude, short-duration polyphasic units. Because of poor muscle function, tension produced by individual motor units is reduced, and many units are recruited to produce a weak contraction.

Normal

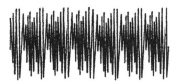

Myopathic

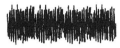

Figure 11-7. A full but low-amplitude recruitment pattern of myopathy. (Courtesy of Seward Rutkove, M.D.)

The EMG signs of myopathy are short-duration, low-amplitude polyphasic units with a complete or full recruitment pattern (Fig. 11-7). The presence of fibrillation potentials at rest suggests an inflammatory or a metabolic dysfunction, such as acid maltase deficiency, among others.

NERVE CONDUCTION STUDIES

Motor Conduction Studies

Transcutaneous electrical stimulation of a motor nerve results in an observable twitch of the muscle that it supplies. The electrical evoked response or compound muscle action potential (CMAP) can be recorded with a surface or needle electrode placed over or in the muscle. Usually, a surface pick-up electrode is used. In the upper limb, the median and ulnar nerves are easily studied in this way. The recording muscle for the median nerve is abductor pollicis brevis, and for the ulnar nerve, abductor digiti minimus.

The median or ulnar nerve is stimulated at multiple points along its course—wrist, axilla, and above and below the elbow. The skin is marked at each stimulus point. A surface stimulating bipolar electrode delivers slow repetitive or single square-wave pulses of current of varying voltage, and the cathode (−) is placed closer to the recording electrode than the anode (+). The stimulus voltage is gradually increased, which results in a graduated increase of the CMAP or M wave as more axons are activated. Ultimately, no further increase is seen, which denotes that a supramaximal stimulus has stimulated the fastest conducting motor fibers of the nerve. On the oscilloscope, a small stimulus artifact marks the point of stimulation, and after a varying latent period, the M wave is seen (Fig. 11-8). The latency from stimulus artifact to the M wave in milliseconds is proportional to the conduction velocity and the distance that the impulse must travel; the

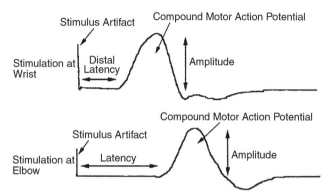

Figure 11-8. Motor conduction study responses. Note that the latency increases with proximal stimulation at the elbow. (Courtesy of Seward Rutkove, M.D.)

latter is measured by referral to the skin markings. The distance between two skin marks in centimeters can now be related to the difference in latency of two stimuli in milliseconds delivered at those points, which allows for calculation of the conduction velocity (CV) between the stimulation points in meters per second. Normal motor CVs for the upper limb muscles are 50–70 m per second.

Usually, the CV increases slightly in more proximal segments of the nerve, but a segmental decrease in CV—that is, segmental slowing—suggests a localized area of demyelination, often due to peripheral entrapment. In the case of median entrapment in the carpal tunnel, the site of nerve compression is distal to the most peripheral stimulation point, and the conduction velocity can therefore not be calculated. In this situation, norms are available for the distal terminal latency, and a prolonged terminal latency indicates a localized demyelinated segment of nerve in the tunnel.

Attention should also be directed to the CMAP. The area of the negative phase of the CMAP is directly proportional to the number of muscle fibers depolarized, but area is difficult to measure, and amplitude serves the same purpose if the duration of the evoked potential is normal. Normal amplitude is 4–20 mv. A low-amplitude CMAP suggests an axonal process, whereas normal amplitude can be seen in the presence of slow conduction, indicating a primarily demyelinating process.

When a nerve is stimulated, the stimulation evokes action potentials that propagate orthodromically toward the muscle, but also antidromically toward the anterior horn cell. Some anterior horn cells are activated to discharge another orthodromic impulse to the muscle. These recurrent discharges produce a small muscle potential or F wave, with a latency of 20–40 ms, depending on the distance from the site of stimulation to the spinal cord

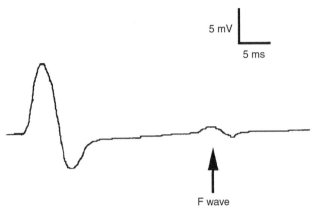

Figure 11-9. The F wave is seen sometime after the M, or compound muscle action potential, wave. (Courtesy of Seward Rutkove, M.D.)

(Fig. 11-9). Because the pathway of F waves is long and traverses both proximal and distal parts of the nerve, including root, their latency gives an indication of conduction over the whole motor pathway. The F wave is delayed in patients with more proximal and also peripheral pathology. If peripheral CV is normal, a delayed F wave supports the notion of plexus or root pathology.

Sensory Conduction Studies

Sensory nerve conduction studies are often more sensitive than motor conduction studies for demon-

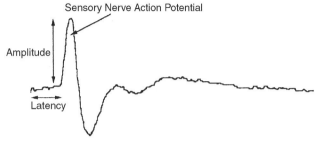

Figure 11-10. Sensory evoked potential. The median nerve was stimulated at the wrist and the evoked potential was recorded at digit two. (Courtesy of Seward Rutkove, M.D.)

strating mild disorders. Orthodromic or antidromic conduction velocities are the same in sensory nerves, and the technique used is that which is most clinically appropriate. Thus, ring electrodes over a finger may be used to stimulate the median or ulnar digital branches with pick-up surface electrodes at the wrist, or the nerve can be stimulated at the wrist and the evoked potential (sensory nerve action potential) can be picked up with finger recording electrodes (Fig. 11-10). Supramaximal stimuli are recorded. The amplitudes are small—in the region of 5–80 μv—and require amplification by way of signal averaging.

The latency to the response is again directly related to the rate of conduction and the distance between stimulating electrodes, as marked on the skin. Slow conduction or an absent sensory nerve action potential indicates neuropathy.

FURTHER READING

Aminoff MJ. Electrodiagnosis in Clinical Neurology. New York: Churchill Livingstone, 1980.

Summary of Treatment Options

The possible options for treatment are best summarized in a flow diagram (Fig. 12-1).

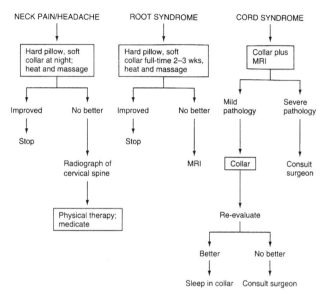

Figure 12-1. Algorithm for the treatment of cervical spondylosis. (MRI = magnetic resonance imaging.) (Reprinted with permission from RT Johnson and JW Griffin. Current Therapy in Neurologic Disease [5th ed]. St. Louis: Mosby, 1996;77.)

Index